Health Relearned

Why Diets, Workouts, and Pills Always Fail

By: Garrett Busch

About Garrett Busch

I am a business owner, health coach, and article contributor to health and fitness outlets. I have extensively studied the field of health and fitness for over seven years now searching for solutions to problems that have plagued not only my clients, but the ones I love the most as well.

I have been a health enthusiast about as far back as I can remember. I was cooking my own recipes at the age of 9 and reading every publication I could get my hands on. Although, my passion for health and quality of life really took off when I was 13. As you will read further in this book, during this time my grandfather had a heart attack at 54 and died. This was followed by other loved ones going through open heart surgeries, cancer treatments, and drastic medical procedures at ages far too young.

I saw a distinct problem and one that wasn't getting fixed. I was caught in the same traps as many of my colleagues early throughout my journey in this crazy industry until I had an epiphany that changed the way I approach my health and my clients.

Poor health has resulted in losses of life, happiness, health, wealth, and fulfillment for a majority of my loved ones. I knew there had to be a better way. I knew this was not and could not be, the "new normal". I became obsessed by my mission to recreate a healthy American society. I used research from historical cultures, modern-day tribes, current countries who are succeeding in this field, and saw common threads for success. I gathered all of the information needed and went to work creating simple strategies and implementations that will force health, happiness, and success through habits.

I can firmly say that I have created a book that I am proud of, a book that I have used to change many lives from clients to family members, and a book that I know will stand the test of time and future research.

I hope you enjoy this book and it truly positively impacts your life. For more information about me or this book you can find me at garrettbusch.com/blog.

Acknowledgements

I would like to thank the following people for their invaluable input

and support during this process.

Britney Bergen

John Xanthos

Tim Moehring

Coreen Busch

Cortney Sutherland

No matter what stage you're at in your health journey, I believe the strategies and interactions in this book will bring you insight to enhance your happiness, health, and quality of life. If you enjoy this book and it has produced benefits in any capacity for your health and life, I would greatly appreciate a review and feedback of any kind. Thank you for supporting this author and the countless hours that have gone into making this effort a reality.

Table of Contents

Chapter 1: Understanding Health in the Big Picture

It is time to realize that in the past, you have been tricked. Have you fallen for *Six-Minute Abs*? Maybe it was whatever xyz diet? A celebrity cleanse or detox? Promises, oh the promises you have been told. Eventually these endless myriads of promises fail and you end up burnt out with lost hope.

Or they lead you down the **rabbit hole**. This diet didn't work, but maybe the next one will! You begin constantly chasing the "new best diet" or the next "amazing fat burning exercise routine". The new trend that is "guaranteeing" your success.

However, for 99% of us these never work. These programs are restrictive, they go against your life, and they only make your daily routine more difficult by forcing you to carve out vast amounts of time and effort. It is time to realize that diets and workouts will never work for the majority of busy Americans. What does work? Micro-habits.

As with anything, we must first start with the why.

Why should you be healthy?

Let me guess....

To have a six-pack?

To look good?

Or to fit into that new dress?

These are the typical responses I hear from people when I ask this question. Unfortunately, health has become a superficial issue. As a performance coach, I used to buy into this trap. I drew excitement out of clients with statements like,

"Let's get you back to your high school weight!"

"Let's drop six inches off your waistline!"

"You're going to look better than you ever have!"

The excitement was there in the beginning. My male clients eagerly showed up week after week, proud to show me the new hole in their belt they conquered. My female clients flaunted their new Lululemon yoga pants that were a couple sizes smaller and fixed with purple, cloud-like shapes. All of my clients were constantly flexing in the ever-reflecting maze of gym mirrors, eyeing the new shadows that appeared from definitions freshly cut into the muscle like a carved stone.

The excitement began to fade as time went on. New routines, new exercises, new diet plans, new workout environments, periodization, you name it, the changes weren't working. The plateaus we experienced were grander than Mt. Kilimanjaro. Ironic. They hovered over us, just waiting to dump an avalanche of fresh powder that would wash away all the progress we had made.

Why did these plateaus occur? Why couldn't we break through them?

It was because as a coach, I was thinking small.

I later read David J. Schwartz's book, *The Magic of Thinking Big*, and discovered my problem. In Schwartz's book, he explains that if you think in large ways, you will have grand accomplishments, but if you think in small ways, your life and accomplishments will also be small. Like my clients, I was thinking small. I was measuring their results in superficial ways without diving any deeper than the artificial surface of appearances.

I'll admit, I was extremely happy seeing a client lose 30 pounds or taking five inches off their waist line. However, I did not factor in the much larger things occurring in their lives: career-changing promotions, getting the girl or guy they desired, or finally feeling happiness.

Then I started to think: what if health and fitness just became a byproduct of the bigger goal? What if I started thinking bigger and went after my clients' life goals right away?

Then it hit me: health isn't about looking good. Health can literally change any and every aspect of your life. This is what the health and fitness industry doesn't always grasp. Coaches are always trying to get x physical results, this mile time or a 305 lb. bench press. *When none of that even matters.*

Did our ancient ancestors exercise, eat well, and create a healthy lifestyle so that they could look at their reflection in a pond and say, "Raawrr, biceps real big, amazing!" No! They exercised, ate well, and created that lifestyle to live, survive, progress the species and enlighten themselves! They focused on what actually matters. These were way bigger than something as trivial as looks. These were primal instincts that our souls demanded satisfaction from. These encompassed our entire lives. *They were our entire lives.*

Today, we don't give a shit about health because we treat it with such a minuscule reward: looking good. Great, now I have a smaller waist and bigger shoulders, now what? Umm, I don't know, let's try to lift heavier weights, eat cleaner, and run faster! Ok, I can run a little faster, I'm eating better, and I can lift a little more weight, now what? Unless you're incredibly vain, this will never completely satisfy you. We are treating health and fitness as singular items, detached from the rest of our lives.

Since this period of discovery, my whole approach to health has changed. I now treat health with the respect it deserves. It isn't a body in the mirror. It isn't a damn diet. It isn't how much weight you can lift. Health is everything you want to accomplish. Health is living a virtuous life full of happiness, love, and wealth. Health is living the life you have always dreamed about.

There is no detachment between health and your goals, they intertwine so delicately that they are impossible to separate.

I now start out by asking my clients, "What are the biggest goals you have for yourself in life?" Not what you want out of fitness and health, but what you want out of life. Their responses are inspiring:

"To grow my business to be a millionaire."

"To live on the beach."

"To get the girl of my dreams."

"To cross everything off my bucket list."

"To finally find my true happiness."

I always respond to this inspiration with, "Ok, this is the first day of achieving those goals and we will achieve those goals."

Health now became that primal instinct again. We were working on our health for something bigger, something actually important, something life-changing.

Those prior plateaus were engulfed by typhoons of determination. I saw my clients' willpower shoot to the stars. We created a "no-other-options" mentality and there was nothing that was going to stop us from accomplishing those goals.

My programs are now exponentially more well-rounded. I go far beyond the typical approach of ineffective diets and workouts; I now focus on habitual changes that ripple through my clients' lifestyles, nutrition, and way of thinking. The results have been staggering and were enough to inspire me to write this book. I no longer wanted to change a handful of client's life's, I wanted to change an entire society, a population. I will change your life.

You want a certain lifestyle? Let's create it. Do you want to finally live the life you were meant for? Let's get to work. These are the first pages to the rest of your life and they have already started. Hop on and enjoy the ride, because you are now on track to accomplish the goals you have always dreamed of.

Some of you will try to skip ahead to get to a secret potion. Most of you are accustom to the snake oil salesman pitching a supplement or diet. The American paradigm: the quick fix. The short cut. The miracle diet. The one pill that cures all! That is not the way this works. Anyone who tells you they have these is *full of shit*.

I am not going to change your life by selling you some bullshit, nor am I going to lie to you. You're going to get uncomfortable. You will discover some things emotionally and mentally that will make you rethink a lot of how you have been living your life. You will learn a lot of factual and scientifically proven information, through cited scientific studies.

In reality, I can't force you to do anything. You have to take the tools and the knowledge I am giving you, along with the strategic implementations I outline, and actually use these every day to create successful habits. The proverb, "Give a man a fish and you feed him for a day. Teach a man to fish and you feed him for a lifetime," stands true here.

I will make it *easier* for you to do them, I will change the way you think, I will change the way you see your goals and yourself, and I will change the way you view your health.

The truth is you already can accomplish your goals. You're completely capable of everything you want, the only thing holding you back is your behaviors. You have the skills, the abilities, the mind, the body, the determination, everything you need to change your life. Your habits have just led you astray.

Together we will change these habits and unlock everything you have dreamed of.

Now is the time to *let your emotions fly*. This is your life! If you truly want a better life, if you know that you're not where you should be, this is the time to let it out. **Write down your goals, then shout them out loud**! *Shout them into the mirror*. Know that we will accomplish these together. I will set you on the right path and you will soon have control over your life. Now put the pen to the paper and let those emotions free…. What will you gain out of life? What will you accomplish? What dreams will you make a reality?

Write down your three most important life goals:

1. _____

_____

_____

_____

Why is this your goal?_____

_____

_____

_____

2. _____

_____

_____

_____

Why is this your goal?_____

_____

_____

_____

3. _____

_____

_____

_____

Why is this your goal?_____

_____

_____

_____

Now it is time to explore the ways we will accomplish your

goals. We will start with the paradigm shift in your psychology that

will change the way you think about everything you do in health and beyond. Next, we will implement *minute* lifestyle habits that will positively help you more than you could ever imagine and lead you straight to your goals. After this, we will discuss basic nutritional guidelines and strategies to make food simple with good habits, not diets. Finally, we will ditch the workouts and make exercise fun again, the way it was throughout your childhood. That is right, contrary to everything you have been lead to believe, exercise can actually be fun.

Now let's get to work and **accomplish your goals**. We will address your personal plateaus, understand why they exist, and correct them with real incentives used in fun and strategic ways to watch your dreams become reality. No more celebrity cleanses that don't do anything but *torture* you and make you *shit water* for two weeks. No 30-day, I'm an asshole at every restaurant, diet. No sweating until we collapse and destroy our joints, CrossFit exercise routine. No bullshit pills claiming to cure our metabolism, unproven through science. Just simple changes.

That.

Actually.

Fucking.

Work.

1.1: Psychology, Lifestyle, Nutrition, and Fitness

When it comes to your health, we need to focus on your mental, emotional, and physical health. Each of these affects the other, and if any one part is missing, it will create an imbalance in your life.

There is a good chance you're fat, unhappy, or unhealthy, and want to change this. I'm not saying this to be arrogant or judgmental, I'm saying this **statistically**.

In 2015, it was reported that 70% of the American population is now either overweight or obese.[1] Countless studies examining everything from cancer rates to happiness to life expectancy, show that being overweight negatively affects your health and life in monumental ways.

Remember, health is more than a body in the mirror. Even if you're skinny you may have very unhealthy habits that are affecting your goals. For example, did you know that 70% of

Americans are unhappy at work?[2] Even worse, more than 30 million Americans are on anti-depressants.[3]

We are not talking about not being happy. We are talking about severe, life-altering depression. A **black-hole** that leaves its' victims with *bloody hands and lost voices*. A **pit** so inescapable those affected feel that they must take a daily pill in order to keep living. 30 million Americans translates to one in every ten men, women, and children in this country. If you narrowed it down to adults ages 22-65, then the ratio becomes increasingly staggering. The statistics don't stop there.....

Close to 70% of American adults are on some form of prescription medicine.[4]

We have all heard that 50% of American marriages end in divorce. Recent research shows this rate is actually closer to 40%, which is still mind-blowing.[5] We are talking about a *marriage*, a *LIFE-partnership*, till *DEATH* do us part.

The average American sits for 13 hours a day.[6]

More than 80% of Americans will experience back pain in their lifetime.[7]

Approximately 50 million Americans live in chronic pain, every, single, day.[8]

More than 133 million Americans have a chronic illness.[9]

Americans average just over six hours of sleep per night.[10]

About 90% of Americans have regrets in their life.[11]

Are you seeing the trends here yet?

We are supposedly living better than anyone ever has in history. Yet, the statistics show this is far from reality.

Our health is getting worse despite our medical care becoming the best it ever has been. We have bigger homes and nicer cars, yet we are still vastly unhappy. We can buy any item online with the click of a mouse on Amazon, yet we are still left unsatisfied. We have indoor plumbing and air conditioning, yet we don't sleep enough and suffer from chronic stress. We sit on our asses all day, yet we wonder why we have chronic pain. We have paid services for everything, unlimited entertainment, and restaurants on demand, but our relationships are failing just as much now, as ever before. Our technology is incredible, yet we are still not living to the fullest. Diseases that didn't exist or were extremely rare 100 years ago are now rampant through our society.

The methods we are using in the health and fitness industry are *failing us*. We put in place restrictive diets and monotonous exercise routines that leave us miserable and bored to tears. We are trying to force health on ourselves through extreme practices. We make health painstakingly organized, which goes against its very nature. We separate our health into meticulously timed one-hour blocks at the gym and count our food down to the calorie and macro. Ridiculous.

None of this is working!

How do I know none of this is working? Because the statistics keep getting worse! Every single year we are getting fatter, unhappier, more unhealthy, and worth less. The millennial generation is the first generation that will live **SHORTER** lives than their parents. We are far from maxing out our longevity or quality of life.

A recent study by the Mayo Clinic shows that *only 2.7%* of Americans meet the *basic* qualifications for a healthy lifestyle.[53] Two. Point. Seven. Percent!

Americans are living in poor health and falling short of accomplishing their goals when it comes to wealth, happiness, and love. Guess what? *It doesn't have to be this way*. It shouldn't be! From now on, for you, IT WILL NOT BE.

Compared to other first-world countries, we are failing when it comes to our health. There are cultures on this Earth today where many of these problems simply do not exist, and we will examine how they are outpacing us in health. What's even more fascinating is that we have all of the solutions to fix these problems. Some of them you may have heard of, others you may be hearing for the first time in this book, but they do exist and are often times so simple!

I will be the first to tell you: I am not amazing.

No not you.

I mean **me**.

Garrett Busch.

The author.

I did not magically invent all of these solutions. Most of them are right in front of our faces. They have existed throughout history and are well-documented through texts and research, both past and present. I have studied these solutions vigorously, day-in and day-out for seven years now. I am so passionate about these issues because they have plagued myself and the ones I love.

My grandfather died at the young age of 54 due to a heart attack. I watched others go through open-heart surgeries and drastic medical procedures due to deteriorating health. I witnessed friends battling depression and anxiety. I saw the ones I love not being able to enjoy life as much as possible.

I realized I was not the person I wanted to be. Constantly lacking focus and energy, sleep deprived, questioning my life. I was plagued by injuries that affected my psyche from the moment I woke up every day. I was not fully giving myself to my significant other. Simply put, I was lacking happiness.

I knew this was not the way I or my loved ones were supposed to live. I refused to believe this was just the *"new normal"*. From here, I set out on my mission to change American health.

I knew we needed to change our health as a nation in order to keep progressing. As a nation we are only as strong as our weakest links and poor health is holding us back. According to the Centers for Medicare & Medicaid Services as of 2015 Americans spend **3.2 TRILLION dollars** on healthcare.[55] That means we spend $10,000 per person every single year on healthcare![55] At the same time, many other countries around the world are beginning to fall into the same unhealthy trap.

If we reverse the health epidemic we will create even more innovation, more advancement, and more opportunity for every American. We can create a country brimming with happiness from Hawaii to Maine and Alaska to Florida. America just needs a spark to get it there and with the passion deep in my heart I set out to be the catalyst for this transformation.

Through my passion, I studied health's history, tribal cultures past and present, other modern cultures, and all of the clinical research that goes with them. I am not some communist hippie who thinks we need to give up our material possessions to live better lives. Health and our goals are not a black and white topic, all or nothing.

The truth is we can live the best of both worlds. We will balance your life and health, while still accomplishing your goals. In fact, it will make accomplishing your goals that much easier and even automatic!

After reading the first paragraphs of this chapter you might be thinking, "Oh great, so he wants me to quit my job and never sit in a chair for the rest of my life." No, stop it, that's not even close. The goal of this book isn't to turn your life upside down with a diet, workout plan, or restrictive lifestyle. There are already tons of these programs that exist and if they actually worked for the majority of people, we wouldn't be in a health epidemic as a country.

On the contrary, I want to make this as **easy** as possible. I want to make these habits so minute that you barely even realize they're happening. By making these changes small-scale I know you will be successful. Good health is attainable for <u>every person</u> on this planet and it will help you accomplish everything you want in life.

Most of this book I want to layout in that big picture format I talked about before. Most of what I'm telling you are strategies and principles, you then have the power to cookie cut them for your life.

There are four main categories of our lives that affect our health: our psychology, lifestyle, nutrition, and fitness. Just like our physical, mental, and emotional health, these four things must work together.

Health is so important because it affects everything that we do and how we act. Typical programs never focus on a well-rounded approach that works with the individual's life. Instead, most programs go against the individual and actually make their life *harder*.

This book is different. We are going to approach health from a full-spectrum view and create healthy habits that enhance your life, not work against you.

You must grasp that health is not a detachable item. Health weaves in and out of your wealth, happiness, and love. If you are unhealthy, you will not have as much wealth as you otherwise could have, your relationships will falter, the love you so crave will suffer, and your overall happiness will dwindle as a result.

People usually look at health in a divided matter. They think of this as only working out or only following a diet, when health interlocks with everything in our lives. By focusing on your mental, physical, and emotional health you will directly and indirectly be setting yourself up for success in those other parts of your life: wealth, happiness, and love. To make sure that we are sufficiently covering every aspect of your health and life, we must examine your psychology, lifestyle, nutrition, and fitness and all of your habits within each of these factors.

Humans are a construct of their daily behaviors. Those behaviors become our habits. From sunup to sundown we string all of our habits together to form the person we are right now. The ways we think and act become automatic. We don't even realize what most of our habits are, let alone how they affect us.

If you become mindful of your habits and continually practice the right habits in each of the four categories above, then you can be confident you **are** going to achieve success.

Now we are getting on the right page. Health isn't about a body. It isn't superficial. It truly impacts every action and thought, throughout your entire life. Let's start with your frame of mind and discover how you can use your thought processes and behaviors to set yourself up for success.

Chapter 2: The Psychology of It All

Our psychology is truly amazing and so is the brain. A powerhouse, an intricate web of thoughts, behaviors, and feelings, encased in a protective, armored skull which continues to puzzle scientists all over the world. Through research, it is more clear that the mind-body connection is very real and more powerful than we ever thought.[44] That is why you can't change your habits without consciously observing them and figuring out what you are doing wrong.

Habits are habits for a reason after all.

When it comes to accomplishing your goals, understanding your psychology can be the difference maker between success and failure. You can physically do everything right, but if you doubt yourself or your goals, you ultimately will not be successful. It is so important to **constantly** remind yourself of your goals and why you want to accomplish them. Never lose sight of why you're making these necessary changes. *Believe in yourself and your* *future*. The more you remind yourself of your goals and envision your success, the more likely you are to succeed.

Let's dive deep into some common pitfalls that keep us from using our minds to their full potential. Now is the time to get involved. Grab the pen you used to write down your goals and be active throughout this discussion.

I want you to note some of the problem areas that you're currently stuck in and the strategies you will use to get out of them. <u>Underline</u>. Write in the margins. **Highlight**. Circle the key takeaways you need the most and use the interactive sections in this book.

This is one of the greatest moments of your life! You're on the cusp of enlightenment and the first step on that journey is to examine your psychology.

Key Takeaways:

- **You must first observe your habits before you can change them.**

- It is critically important to constantly remind yourself of your goals, why you want to accomplish those goals, and to envision your success.

2.1: Controlling the Mind

We have to realize how powerful the mind is. Your mind and the way you think, can make or break you and your entire life. I remember my sister had a concert recital in the 10th grade; she played the violin. I desperately did not want to go, because I'd rather be playing video games or watching TV, the life of an average teenager. My parents told me, "Too bad, you're going."

As a child would, I acted pissed off and angry the whole ride there. Frivolous pouting: the melody of a 12-year-old. Once there, my Dad took me aside and told me, "You can make this the best night of your life or the worst, you have all of the power and are making all of the decisions."

At first, in my little child mind, I thought, "Screw you, you dragged me here, I have no power."

Later, we went into the recital and boredom kicked in. Negativity after all, is boring. A shallow hole filled with the same lambasting thoughts, *both futile and draining*. That boredom lasted all of five minutes before I thought to myself, "What's so bad

about this?"

I couldn't really think of anything. It was something new,

interesting, I'd never been before, and the music was actually

pretty nice to listen too.

Just like that, my dad's words seared into my mind and I

decided to try to make it the **best** night of my life.

Happiness on the other hand is *riveting*, one hundred

thousand Christmas lights synergistically illuminating beauty at the

flick of a switch. The senses coming alive and awakening the soul.

In the instance of a subtle change, the string quartet that was

Irvine High School became vibrant in the glow of immaculate

chandeliers. Their music created a whimsical energy that pulsed

with every heartbeat. Each note beautifully crisp. Every crescendo

spiking adrenaline levels.

Now, I can't definitively say that night was better than telling

my girlfriend I loved her for the first time or that amazing nighttime snow walk I had in Quebec City on vacation. Regardless, I can tell you I will *forever* remember the recital and how happy I was to see my sister play the violin.

The way we think can determine every action we take throughout our entire lives. Have you ever wondered why the majority of unsuccessful people are unhappy and pessimistic, and the majority of successful people happy and optimistic?

It's not a coincidence.

It's not random.

It is not because of what they have.

Their wealth and happiness are simply byproducts of their habits; not the other way around.

There are countless scientific studies showing negativity is actually, physically, **killing us.**[12] Negativity weakens your immune system, builds stress, raises your blood pressure, and releases a plethora of cortisol, the stress hormone, which slowly but surely cripples your body and mind.[12] The result of this is an

immeasurable loss of wealth, health, happiness, and love.

On the contrary, there are recent studies involving the use of CAT

scans which show Buddhist monks with happiness activity levels in

the brain that are unseen in Western society.[13] These results are

fascinating when you consider these monks live relatively simple

lives with few materials.

The Bhagavad Ghita sums it up by saying along the same lines,

your mind can be your best friend or your worst enemy. This is a

scripture over 5100 years old that science is now starting to

confirm through studies.

This is not a coincidence.

It's time you start living your life to the fullest. Let's examine

how you currently think, how this negatively affects your goals,

and how you can change your negative psychology.

Key Takeaways:

- You have all of the power to make every day or situation the best or worst one of your life.

- Negativity is scientifically proven to physically kill us.

- Your frame of mind can make or break any goal you have and your success in life.

2.2: Ditching Negativity for a Positive Life

To change your mindset, you need to first understand how you got here. Why are you fat, unhappy, unhealthy, or all three? Now stop…. because I know what is coming next: **excuses**.

Perhaps you could have psychological excuses of early childhood trauma, bullying, substituting food for happiness.

Maybe you have everyday excuses like, "I'm always busy." We will deal with everyday excuses throughout this book and completely eliminate these by changing your habits.

However, when it comes to dealing with the past we must take a different approach. We need to treat the past as a *sunk cost*. In economic terms, a sunk cost is a cost that has already occurred and is irretrievable. If you think of your past as a sunk cost, then everything in your past is already gone and irretrievable. Shut the door, lock the box, and stop dwelling on the past.

Let me be clear: there is a difference between reflecting on the past and dwelling on the past. Reflection is a great tool to bring understanding to your past and use it in a positive way. There is a time to reflect, through either meditation and alone time (which we will talk about later) or a licensed therapist. Both are fantastic and I encourage them.

Successful people use the past as a tool, and they use it seldom. Unsuccessful and negative people dwell on the past, use it as an excuse, and *never let it go*. You have to come to grips that the past is gone. Treat it as the sunk cost that it is and do not let it interrupt your life or way of thinking.

Now I understand this is not exactly easy, especially for someone who has been locked into this habit for years. A great way to get yourself out of this box, is to practice meditation or see a licensed therapist: confront it head on and take it day by day.

For all of your waking hours, you need to change your frame of mind. I know, I know, easier said than done. However, an easy solution which has shown great success is to substitute the negative thoughts with positive ones. Whenever you think of your past negatively, immediately think of two positive things that you're currently doing to get closer to your goals.

Two positive thoughts could be, "I'm really happy I took a 10-minute walk this morning and got in five minutes of meditation, sticking to this routine is getting me that much closer to my first million dollars."

Your praise might be general as, "I'm proud of myself for setting my goals and sticking to the process: I'm on the right path."

Even if you have a random negative thought after someone cut you off on the freeway or you were scolded at work, immediately think of *anything positive*, such as, "It really is a beautiful day outside."

Yes, this is corny.

But yes, <u>this does work</u>.

The more you think negatively, the more the synapses in your brain will be wired to instinctively go towards negative thoughts.[12]

When you think negatively, you become a negative person, which negatively affects your wealth, happiness, and goals.

When you gravitate towards positive thoughts, a whole realm of positive opportunities and experiences await you. Plus, how easy is this to do?

How much energy does it take to formulate a positive thought? It takes almost none. You have complete control over this, so why not do it? Formulating positive thoughts whenever you have a negative thought will make a huge impact in the way you think and view life. It will even change how you think about yourself.

If you understand negativity is a **disease**, forever looking for the vulnerable stitch in your armor, then you're taking the first step to changing your outlook. Negativity is a virus, it travels like the **black plague**, jumping from cell to cell and thrusting its presence into every fiber of your existence.

Think about how negative we and our society have become.

Don't believe me? Turn on the news:

Murder.

Car crashes.

War.

Fire.

Obesity.

Death.

Or, go on social media:

Passive-aggressive friends.

Cyber bullying.

Worrying about what others think.

Superiority complexes.

When something goes wrong in your life, do you always think of the worst case scenario? If your car broke down, would your first thoughts immediately go to, "OMG, my life is over, worst day of my life, my day is ruined,"?

We have all had these thoughts, but we can change these into positives.

Think, is your car breaking down really the worst day of your life?

A broken down car is no doubt an inconvenience but you have to learn to deal with it positively. What do you have to do now that your car is broken down? Walk a little more or ride a bike. Maybe you ask a close friend for a ride the next couple of days. You can commute with your significant other and enjoy some extra quality time. These alternatives would add some extra activity to your day, promote a healthier lifestyle, and help you strengthen a bond with a friend or loved one via some new memories and good conversation. Those are *positives*, not negatives.

I guess this means your life is not really over. In actuality, most people will let a broken down car ruin their day: they will be pissed off for a couple days, complain about the situation to everyone they know, and create stress throughout their whole body *for no reason*. It is incredible how choosing to be positive or negative can impact a couple days of your life so differently. This is how powerful the mind is!

Your mind, the way you think, and your attitude, are everything. <u>Never forget this</u>. You must become a positive person through your own thoughts and actions. You must also cut out the negativity.

Jim Rohn, a famous motivator and entrepreneur, once said, "You are the average of the five people you spend the most time with." I will go even further to say you are the average of the most prominent nouns in your life. We live in a time period where we are often surrounded by technology and materials, more than people. You must be honest with yourself and examine which parts of your life are causing unnecessary negativity.

To get a better picture of what affects you the most day-by-day, make a list below of the ten most influential nouns in your life: nouns are people, places, or things. Next to each noun, write down the positive and negative emotions you experience from each noun.

Prominent Nouns	Positives	Negatives
1. _____	_____	_____
	_____	_____
	_____	_____
2. _____	_____	_____
	_____	_____
	_____	_____
3. _____	_____	_____
	_____	_____
	_____	_____
4. _____	_____	_____
	_____	_____
	_____	_____

5. _____   _____   _____

                     _____   _____

                     _____   _____

6. _____   _____   _____

                     _____   _____

                     _____   _____

7. _____   _____   _____

                     _____   _____

                     _____   _____

8. _____   _____   _____

                     _____   _____

                     _____   _____

9. _____   _____   _____

                     _____   _____

                     _____   _____

10. _____   _____   _____

                     _____   _____

_____   _____

Compare how many positive and negative emotions you experience from each noun. Are there some nouns that are predominately negative?

Do you have a friend who is constantly negative, bitching about everything and everyone in existence?

Do you have a parent who always talks down to you and makes you feel inferior?

Is your social media causing you stress and anxiety?

Do you waste too much of your time constantly checking emails or watching television?

Do you have a job that is beating you down day after day?

Are Websites or games wasting your energy and causing irritability in your relationship?

Are you stuck in a living situation in which you are influenced by others who are making bad choices and doing bad things?

I know many of these prominent negative nouns because I have made this list multiple times and experienced many of the same things as you. Each and every one of your prominent nouns which cause you negative emotions are preventing you from accomplishing your goals.

These negative people, places, and things are affecting the way you think and act. You should be proud of yourself for looking at your environment and dissecting what is affecting you. This is a monumental step. However, the next hurdle is an even taller one.

You must find a way to get rid of your negative emotions or possibly cut the cord and get that noun out of your life.

If your negative emotions outweigh the positives, then it is time for a change. Come to grips that while you may love that noun, if it causes you negative emotions then you need a temporary or permanent break to live a more positive life.

If going cold turkey is too drastic of a change, try setting up short specific timeframes you spend with those nouns, but don't go past those time limits. If the noun begins causing you negative emotions, then their time is up for the day.

Let's use one of the examples from above. Let's say your mother always wanted you to be a doctor. You, on the other hand, wanted to be an artist, teacher, or any other profession. If your mother belittles your profession, you may have to confront her and explain to her that her negative comments about your career are bringing you down. Then explain that if she is negative towards your career, you can't be around her because there are more constructive things you could be doing.

You can explain to her the physical, mental, and emotional consequences of her negativity. If this doesn't get through to her, then every time she brings up how she wishes you were a doctor, then it's simply time for you to go and spend time with another prominent noun that is helping you get closer to your goals.

Be honest with your prominent nouns!

Encourage change, but in the end if that person, place, or thing creates backlash towards you then know it is time to step away. Take a temporary break until that noun can prove to you it is going to contribute to your wealth, health, happiness, and love. If that person or object never brings you closer to your goals, then you may have to dump them or it forever.

Who knows, you may even encourage positive change in that noun. Something as simple as telling a friend their negative gossip isn't helping you or them, may make your friend realize their own negative behavior and help them change for the better. This energy would be better spent talking about two positive experiences that have occurred in your lives.

By writing down that you aren't happy with your job, this could be the first step in creating a plan to realizing your entrepreneurial dreams. If you stopped dwelling on the negatives of your current job and began positively constructing a plan for change, your whole outlook on life could instantly improve.

You only have one life. If you live your life in an environment full of negativity, gossip, and stress, then the outcome of your life will certainly reflect these negative emotions. Become a positive person, surround yourself with positive thoughts and people, and you will be amazed at the outcome.

Key Takeaways:

- **Use meditation or therapy to reflect on your past and use it as a tool for your success.**

- **Always think of two positive thoughts after you have any negative thought.**

- **Remember your most prominent nouns, how they affect you, and get the predominantly negative ones out of your life.**

2.3: Thinking of Health in the Right Way

We are starting to think about life in a positive way; this is a big step! Next, we are going to embrace the paradigm shift in the way we think about our health.

Health is normally thought of as uncomfortable, hard, and inconvenient. We are going to change this to make it exciting, an adventure, and manageable.

Thinking about health in a negative way is an unfortunate issue that has been ingrained in our minds since childhood. We are constantly told being healthy is miserable! Healthy food is gross. Exercise is brutal and will crush you. It takes too much of a time commitment to be healthy.

These lies about health have spread contagiously throughout our society. Sadly, we hear many of these false statements from the ones we look up to the most. These *stigmas* have created a culture so resistant to health that we now take every route possible to avoid a healthy lifestyle. You need to change that mindset because that's all it is: **a mindset**.

Remember the violin recital example? You can always create two outcomes of the same scenario, whether it is a positive outcome or a negative one. Let's take cooking for example.

Cooking can be the most miserable, tasteless experience of your life. Or, it could be an incredible adventure in which you increase your palate and explore new foods, all while being unbelievably proud of creating nutritious meals that will be enjoyable for your family and friends! *That is all up to you.*

If you read that last passage and thought, "Yea easy for you, but you don't have my schedule, blah, blah, fucking blah." Excuses. If you continue to make excuses, you will stay exactly how you are.

On the other hand, if you read the cooking example and said to yourself, "You know, what this could be fun! I've never tried to explore my full capabilities in the kitchen, and I don't even know what dragon fruit coconut curry tastes like," then you're on the right track.

You should observe what kind of reactions you're having while reading this. If you're experiencing negative reactions, take active measures to change those into positive reactions instead.

Let's start with another small shift in the way we think about nutrition.

Unfortunately, advertising and marketing has distorted the way we interpret food in America. We are constantly bombarded with fast food and soda ads. We would view food much differently from our childhood and beyond if all of these ads were replaced with mini cooking commercials using fresh produce and protein to create delicious meals.

Sadly, this probably won't happen anytime soon. A guy can dream, right? In the meantime, you can change the way you view food if you take control of your own mindset. You can do this with a *simple* trick.

Every time you call something a healthy food, say: "Oops, I meant a **good food**."

Every time you call something edible a regular food or food, there is a good chance this is a processed piece of garbage like fast food, chemical and dye-ridden desserts, unhealthy snacks, soda products or something along these lines. We will start calling these heavily processed foods: "Shitty foods."

Or if you prefer not to curse, "Crappy foods" or "Bad foods."

Eventually, you will convert your mind into actually knowing what is good food and what is shitty or bad food, simply by repeating these phrases and categorizing food correctly.

Soon, this way of thinking will be *natural*. You will crave good, nutritious, healthy staples, and you won't even want to touch bad, gross, unhealthy crap foods. In the nutrition section of this book, we will examine which foods are in which category, enabling you to put this plan into action.

These tricks are known by those familiar with Ivan Pavlov, a notable psychologist, as conditioning. Conditioning is a behavior process that occurs when a response becomes predictable as a result of constant reinforcement. With the food example above, we are creating predictable responses to certain foods by constantly reinforcing the correct descriptions of those foods.

These responses then become habits when performed repeatedly.

With most of the psychological, lifestyle, nutritional, and fitness strategies in this book we are conditioning the way your mind views these categories by making small changes and forcing them to become habits by doing them repeatedly.

After performing these healthy actions, it is important to positively reinforce them. Be proud of yourself and your changes! Smile! Sing your own praises, because you're now enacting the right strategies to accomplish your goals.

If you condition your mind to view health differently and positively reinforce yourself every time you do this, you will positively change the way you view your health, your goals, and yourself. It is very easy to change your thoughts and actions if you finally realize you can.

Yes, you can! If you practice the strategies and implementations in this book you will create the habits that will change your life. By doing this you will create a life that enhances your psychology, nutrition, lifestyle and fitness **like a boss**.

Key Takeaways:

- **Think of health in a positive light and get excited about using your health to accomplish your goals.**

- **Use Conditioning to instill good, healthy habits and positively reinforce yourself when you perform those habits.**

2.4: It Actually is Your Fault

What is America's favorite game?

No, not baseball or football. The **blame game**! America loves to play the blame game: we see this in news coverage, channel after channel on television, and we even do it ourselves to the people we care about most.

Take politics for example. Our politicians rarely take responsibility for their actions. It's always the left's fault or the right's, the illegal immigrants' fault you don't have a better job, blame taxes for your lack of or lesser wealth.

Holy shit, it never stops.

Have you ever heard a senator proclaim, "You know, I regret passing this bill, I take full responsibility for it, and I would like to do something to reverse it right now…."? Yeah, I didn't think so.

Unfortunately, this natural reaction to deflect responsibility and play the blame game has crept into our society and become every day practice. I've done it myself and see so many of my loved ones caught up in the practice. It almost becomes the first line of defense when anything goes wrong.

"Well, I wouldn't have forgotten my wallet if you would have grabbed the takeout boxes!" Sound familiar?

This game is toxic. While you can't control how others act, you can start with yourself. You need to take responsibility for your actions. This is so instrumental to creating a positive psychology; however, so overlooked. Why do you eat fast food? Let me guess...

"I have to because I don't have time to cook."

"I have a family."

"I don't know how to cook."

"Fast food is cheap."

You know what these answers reflect? Excuses. YOU can control what you put in your body and your family's bodies. YOU can control how you fuel your body. YOU can choose to cook healthy, good foods instead of sitting in a drive-through line mulling over which shitty food you'll eat in your car. YOU need to realize that by making excuses, you're playing the blame game. You're blaming your surroundings for YOUR poor health decisions.

How does the average person spend their time? Do they go home and spend the remaining five hours of their day talking and learning with their family or being productive?
Most likely, no.

The average person spends the majority of those remaining five hours watching TV, looking on the internet, and ultimately, being lazy.

If you're the family-person-of-the-year or the always-productive-person, good for you: you are the minority. However, even these people need to invest in themselves and you could look at cooking as a stress reliever, a way of creating necessary nutritious fuel that will help complete a project sooner, or as a way to spend quality time with your family while doing something fun.

If you don't try to cook, you can only blame your health problems on yourself.

Stop making excuses and putting the blame on something or someone else.

Why did you have a heart attack? No, do not blame it on the long hours you had to work. Do not blame it on anything else besides yourself.

You did not invest in yourself.

You did not take care of yourself.

You still are not taking responsibility for your actions, simple as that.

Most people will automatically make excuses rather than take responsibility for their own actions. You can change this mindset: all you have to do is make our decisions **relatable** and **personal**.

Why don't you drink water instead of soda? Water is usually free, it is always more accessible, and it is much better for you. You choose soda because you are not taking responsibility for your health. You say, "One soda won't matter," or "But it's only one soda." Every soda matters, especially if it allows you to continue making excuses.

If you do the same thing day after day, it's not just one soda anymore. It is usually about 45 gallons a year for the average American![14] Change this! All you need to do is start taking responsibility for your actions and embedding all of your decisions into your goals.

Make it personal! Stop asking, "Is one soda really that bad?" Instead ask yourself, "Is one soda going to help me lose 20 lbs. this year?" That's good, but remember think *bigger,* embed your decisions into your largest goals.

Ask yourself, "Is this soda going to help me acquire that *Southern California beach house*?"

After embedding your everyday decisions into your life goals, perform them and positively reinforce your actions. Every time you choose to drink water say to yourself, "Hey that wasn't such a big deal, I'm that much closer to accomplishing my goal."

Own every action that you perform, embed each action into your goals, and continue to create positive reinforcements of encouragement when you complete them. Practice this good habit every day and I promise it will change much more than your health.

Practicing a "no excuses mindset" and getting rid of the blame game will make you aware of all your actions and how they affect you. Before you probably never asked yourself that question about the soda or put pressure on yourself to do the right thing.

Implementing these healthy habits will make you accountable and responsible for everything in your life, from your relationships to your career, and it will ultimately make you invest in yourself.

Key Takeaways:

- **End the cycle of the blame game by taking responsibility of your actions and making your decisions both relatable and personal.**

- **Embed every decision you make into your goals and create positive reinforcement when you perform them.**

2.5: Investing in Myself?

Investing in yourself is such a foreign topic to most of us. We are constantly told to invest in our retirement accounts, our homes, our kids, and our belongings, but no one ever tells us to invest in ourselves!

Most of us become rat racers, constantly working jobs we don't particularly like, not living out our dreams, and obstructing our *real goals* for the next iPhone, house, car, or small promotion. When that material item doesn't satisfy us, we rat race towards the next small object and so forth. In reality, investing in yourself will lead you to all of those materials objects and your real goals, faster than rat racing towards them.

I want to go into human history, because ownership and materialism are very new concepts to our species. The modern human species has been around for almost a couple hundred thousand years now.[39] Owning property is the most significant form of ownership and has only been around for a few thousand years, only *a fraction of our species' lives*. It is understandable that this would happen as we settled down, lived longer, and formed societies.

On the other hand, materialism and conspicuous consumption are extremely new. Only in the last 50 to 100 years have they really boomed.

Now I'm not some communist against material goods, I love the style of my Ford Fusion and the fact that my sectional sofa from Ashley Furniture has cloud-like properties when it comes to comfort. Nonetheless, we should realize that materialism is a very new concept and many of us don't know how to deal with it. Not knowing how to deal with it is what leads us to become rat racers.

You must understand the next material is ***not*** going to make you happy, at least not in the long term. Material items can provide us some level of pleasure, but they can't be the focal point of our happiness and ultimately we need balance.

Throughout history, what have been some of the common denominators of happiness and health? Purpose, fulfillment, and enlightenment, just to name a few.

Why has health been so fulfilling throughout our species' history? Because our health was our purpose: reproducing and surviving so that our species could live on. Our ancestors used fitness, nutrition, and their lifestyle as a way to nourish their bodies, keep them active, and continue their mission.

In addition, how did health lead to enlightenment? In every historical culture, fitness, nutrition, and a balanced lifestyle were used to enhance spirituality; for our ancestors to become one with themselves and master their bodies. They had ceremonies to celebrate their well-being, the Earth they were given, and to dive deeper into their consciousness. They practiced meditation to get to know themselves on a deeper level. These ancient cultures used food as a spiritual form of thanking a higher being for strengthening their bodies and providing them energy. They reveled in the abilities of their bodies and regularly tested them. None of these practices were as elementary as materials. These all had enormous meaning. Our ancestors were always thinking big.

Materials go back to thinking small.

Thinking small is thinking about the next car or new television you can buy. Thinking big is passing a business down to the next generation, following your passion and doing something great that will help society, or becoming the best version of yourself, which will help you be a better father, mother, spouse, or friend. The best way to accomplish all of these meaningful paths in life is to invest in yourself just like our ancestors did.

When I quit my job at the bank and decided I wanted to start positively changing peoples' lives through health full-time, I got a large mix of reactions. Almost every question I received revolved around short-term monetary gains.

"But you won't make as much money as you did at the bank!"

"What about saving for retirement next month?"

I talked to a friend one day after he was done with work and he asked me, "Aren't you sad that you didn't make the $300 dollars today that you would have made if you were still working at the bank?"

I simply asked him, "What did you do today at work and what will you do with the rest of your day?"

He then replied, "Well I came in this morning, went through my emails, started typing in customer information into the CRM database, went through customer notes to see if there were any issues that should be escalated, then made some calls to customers to check in and see how we were doing, pretty much the same thing I do every day."

"Ok, great", I replied. "And what will you do at home now that you're done with work?"

He hesitated, knowing where I was going with this. Then he stated, "I'll probably go get a sub sandwich from Publix (the grocery store), then go home, look at Facebook and watch some TV until I have to go to bed."

I then asked if he had learned anything that day or thought he grew as a person. To which he replied, "*No.*"

He quickly came back with a rebuttal, "But most people don't."

And he was right, **most people don't**.

I said, "Well, I didn't make as much money today, but I was able to research spinal disc pathologies and rehabilitation protocols for a recovering athlete I'm training, I read some Tao philosophy and spent some time meditating. I devoted several hours to my book and I worked out at the park while enjoying some nature. Tonight, I will cook an amazing, nutritious meal with a new recipe I found, spend some quality time talking with my girlfriend, and then I will read about sentence variation techniques to create a more exciting narrative for my book."

What did all of these things have in common? I was investing in myself. I was taking care of myself and my health so that I could grow other aspects of my life.

I wasn't worried about trading my time for stagnate income or mindless entertainment, instead I was giving myself the tools necessary so that I could grow as a person and **build the life I wanted**. This isn't some superiority complex, "I'm better than you because I did these things," because I'm not special, <u>everyone should be doing this</u>.

If you are fat, unhealthy, and unhappy, be honest with yourself! How much time do you use daily to truly invest in yourself? Write down how many minutes or hours per day you use to invest in yourself.

_____ Minutes/Hours *Invested*

Next, write down the amount of time during your day that is wasted on meaningless items that do not contribute to your goals. Consider how much time you spend on mindless television, social media, the internet, day-dreaming, gossiping, sitting around doing

nothing, etc.

_____ Minutes/Hours **Wasted**

Analyze this ratio. Is it a good starting point or one that needs

a lot of work? Do you waste the majority of your time online and in

front of a screen? Are you spending ample time being active,

learning or working on your hobbies, spending _quality time_ with

family and friends, researching more about your professional field,

or taking time to relax, unwind, and meditate?

If you spend all of your time doing the former, this will leave

you empty, unhappy, and unfulfilled. If you invest in yourself you

will learn, grown, and find enlightenment. This will lead you to

acquiring much more wealth, health, happiness, and love over the

course of your life.

Everything is a balance of course. Spending time watching a

little television is okay and can be a good stress reliever, but it

shouldn't take up the majority of your time.

You need to invest in yourself while also taking responsibility for your actions and embedding your goals into your actions. Next time you turn on the television ask yourself:

Should I be doing this right now?

Have I spent too much time doing this?

Am I investing in myself and getting closer to my goals?

If you are wasting too much time, then consider cooking dinner instead of waiting until it is too late and settling for fast food. Try to get some activity in or read before you become too tired. You could take a walk with a friend or loved one to talk about your day before it is too dark.

If you find yourself wasting time, simply do anything else that is investing in yourself and getting you closer to your goals.

An easy strategy to invest more in yourself is to have a few go-to activities that you will do whenever you find yourself wasting time. This is a shortcut list. So whenever you do say, "You know what? I am wasting time..... So what should I do instead?" You now have an easy list you can go straight to instead of brainstorming, trying to decide, wasting more time, and most likely staying on the couch.

Name three go-to activities you will do to invest in yourself:

1. _____

_____

2. _____

_____

3. _____

_____

Stop treating health as a waste of time or inconvenience. If you want to become healthy, which will vastly improve your life and help you accomplish any goal you want, then you have to devote some of your time to health and treat health as an investment in yourself for your other goals.

We often think of cooking and exercising as inconveniences, things *"we have to do."* When I ask a friend to take a walk they usually groan. They say, "But we could be watching another episode of this show instead." Health is not a trade-off, neither is investing in yourself, or growing a friendship.

These should be enjoyable things that you recognize as actions that are bettering your life, not making your life harder. By embedding health within your goals and realizing how it affects those goals, this shift will occur. Eventually, you will respect your health and give it the time it deserves.

What is the one thing that will determine your longevity? It is not your income level. It is not how many possessions you own.... IT'S YOUR HEALTH. Why wouldn't you invest in this as much as possible? There is no reason not to! You just have to make it a priority.

Don't think of investing in your health as taking time away from other things, like making money. That is like the freshman college student who thinks they have to cram non-stop for an exam with an all-nighter. What that student learns later is that they will always be better off taking study breaks to meditate, exercise, cook, and sleep. It has been proven through research that by taking these breaks, the student will remember more material and do better on the test, even if they spent less time studying.[54] As I'm sure many of us have learned through experience.

The mind and body need variety and stimulation through many different mediums, not just studying. The same is true for life, work, and leisure.

If you treat life like a rat race, your health will suffer which will cause your relationships to falter, your happiness to dwindle, and your wealth will be far less than you set out for.

<u>Health affects everything</u>. If you don't invest in your health, you are making it much more difficult to accomplish what you want in every other facet of your life. As with everything, always think *bigger*. Understand that you are not just investing in yourself right now, you are investing in your **future**.

Investing in yourself on a daily basis will set you up for everything you want to accomplish in your life. You are a work-in-progress, but by actively investing in that work, you are ensuring that when the opportunities you seek arise, you will be ready for them!

Key Takeaways:

- **Chase your goals, don't get side tracked by the next material item.**

- **Investing in yourself on a daily basis is really investing in your future and preparing you to be ready for any opportunity that comes your way.**

2.6: The $75 Billion Dollar Question

How much do you value your body? Think of a specific dollar amount right now and write it down:

I _____ (your name) value my body at $ _____.

What if I told you I would make you the richest person in the world, after taxes of course, but if you accepted this money, you would be paralyzed from the neck down. Would you take it? *Not a chance in* **Hell**.

I have never met anyone who would say yes to this agreement and even if someone did accept it, they would surely regret it in the near future.

With that said, congratulations! You just valued your body at over 75 billion dollars. That is a substantial sum of money in our modern world, thus you value your body very highly.

However, if you really value your body so highly, why are you fat, unhealthy, unhappy or all of the above? There are many reasons, but for starters, you are probably thinking about short term trade-offs instead of the long-term outcomes.

In a Stanford experiment by psychologists Walter Mischel and Ebbe B. Ebbesen, children were given two options: (1) get one marshmallow now or (2) wait 15 minutes and get *two* marshmallows. Only a third of the children were able to hold out for the two marshmallow reward. Why you ask? Instant gratification vs. delayed gratification.

This is a perfect example of American culture as a whole. We all want things immediately, even if they're not the best for us. That is why we struggle to save for retirement. In the food industry, this is why so many of us resort to eating out at fast food restaurants or restaurants in general, instead of cooking. We don't like to exercise because we can't see immediate benefits of muscle growth or weight loss after one workout.

If we value instant gratification, we then have trouble investing in ourselves. We often don't see that if we take 30 minutes of our day to invest in ourselves through meditation, food prep, or exercise, that over time this will make us healthier, more successful, and happier: aka delayed gratification.

Often times we only see 30 minutes of the day that could have been used to do something else, usually online or through a television: instant gratification. You need to decide whether you will use those 30 minutes for instant gratification, or delayed gratification that actually builds yourself and your future.

We also have a hard time distinguishing upfront costs vs. long-term costs. In a financial sense, health does not always distinguish itself in dollars until it is too late. I could take on a client and change their nutrition, fitness, lifestyle, and psychology with many alternatives that will only make their life more enjoyable.

Although, sometimes those clients only see the upfront cost of $150 per week in personal training sessions, $50 per week in extra grocery costs, and the time necessary to accomplish these lifestyle and psychological changes. These clients don't always immediately understand the long-term benefits:

You will save money by cooking at home more often.

You will have a sense of accomplishment and be proud of yourself.

You will be setting a good example for your children, family, and friends.

The positive change in your frame of mind will make your business and career more successful.

You will acquire more income and happiness by investing in yourself.

You will become emotionally empowered and more available to your loved ones with an improvement in your health.

All of these will lead to more success and a greater fulfillment of life. Start thinking of the big picture! Think about the next 5, 10, and 30 years, not tomorrow or 30 minutes from now. If the positive reinforcement isn't enough, think about the negatives.

Now we are talking about **real tangible losses,** long-term costs:

Laying in a coffin **twenty years** too soon.

Missing out on your grandchildren's accomplishments.

Losing Tens of thousands of dollars on medical bills.

Not having the energy to experience life to the fullest.

Not accomplishing the goals you always wanted to achieve.

Other's having a **negative perception** of you, which may lead

to **lost opportunities and wealth**.

Starting to get the big picture? Health is more than just

looking good. Once again, we are reminded that health

encompasses not only our mind, body, and spirit, but also our

wealth, happiness, love, and success. Those unhealthy short cuts of

laziness, poor lifestyle habits, shitty food, and damaged thinking

will sideline your goals slowly but surely.

You need to continue to make health a focal point in your

goals. If you correlate the strength of your health with the likelihood of accomplishing your life goals, you will be much more motivated to make the necessary changes.

You have to continue to pound it into your consciousness how much you value your health and always remember that the delayed gratification of accomplishing your goals, will be so much sweeter than the short cuts right in front of you that are steering you away. Fill in the blanks:

I _____ (your name) value my body at $75,000,000,000 and know the long-term success of accomplishing the following goals _____

_____

_____

_____

_____

will **always** be better than the short-term trade-offs that give short-lived instant gratification.

If you're always in pain and tired, you won't do your best work. If your energy levels are always teetering on crashing not only will your productivity and career suffer, but so will your social life. You won't go out to as many events as you could. You probably won't have sex as often as you should with your significant other.

Even if you do it definitely won't be any of the good sex, you know what I'm talking about! Missionary after jeopardy, just going through the motions with your mind wandering off, waiting to be done vs. pulse racing, dripping sweat, warm breath on your shoulder giving you chills, sensitive to every touch, using every wall and piece of furniture in sight as a prop....

We all know the difference. Ergo, with the former, it should be of no surprise if that relationship falters. Which brings more stress, more anxiety and more worrying about the future. Eventually we fall behind at work, becoming lazier and filling with self-pity which decreases our health even more. And the rabbit hole continues.

Spiraling into descent.

Soon you will look back and wonder what happened to all those years:

Why didn't I enjoy life as much as possible?

When did my relationship become so dull?

When did my goals become such a *distant memory*?

All because you took the instant gratification and created short-term tradeoffs.

Thinking small won't get us out of this funk and the instant gratification will fade when we don't see immediate effects. However, implementing health back into your goals will set you on the path for success. *Reverse engineer* it if you have to: deconstruct every step of what you're doing and relate it back to your goals.

Start with the goal and trace it back to your current action, "My business is going to profit two million dollars this year, because I will take responsibility for my actions. My relationship with my wife will not be a distraction and will actually motivate me to do my best work. This will happen by having more vigor, being present in the moment, and getting back to a healthier sex life. These actions will start by eating better today, being slightly more active, and having a positive mindset so that I will have the energy to set of all of these things in motion and accomplish my goal."

Reverse engineering and deconstructing your actions gives you a different perspective of the events unfolding.

No matter what trick you use, always remember the delayed gratification will be worth the wait. Keep reminding yourself that you're on track to accomplish your goals. Keep thinking big! Know that your healthy actions are getting you closer to the life you want.

Things don't happen overnight, so don't be discouraged if you don't see results immediately in any of your practices. You are not rat racing. You are not working towards next week or even next month. You are working towards your *entire future*. Don't let your goals out of your sight and continually seek the habits that will lead you to success.

Key Takeaways:

- **Continually remind yourself that your body is worth $75,000,000,000 and that the delayed gratification of accomplishing your goals will always be better than the short-term tradeoffs.**

- **Remember how large your tangible losses are and the long-term benefits which await you as a result of your healthy habits.**

- **Reverse engineering and deconstructing your actions can help you reinforce good habits.**

2.7: Learned Helplessness is Killing You

Psychologists Martin Seligman and Steven F. Maier discovered the concept "learned helplessness" accidentally.

I won't go into detail about the whole experiment and how they shocked dogs to get their results, this was the 1960's mind you and research ethics were a little different back then. However, the research results from this famous experiment and how they have been used since is fascinating.

In essence, learned helplessness is a **learned behavior** that occurs when someone believes they are powerless. This actually does occur in our modern lives and is probably more prevalent now than ever before in history because we don't seek out the answers to our own problems.

How many times have you asked a boss, parent, or peer a question and right after you heard the answer you thought, "Oh, I knew that!" You have just demonstrated learned helplessness to a degree. You knew the answer, you could have figured it out, but you became helpless and relied on someone else to perform the action for you or tell you the answer to your problem.

When a person demonstrates learned helplessness over and over they start making it a habit. Some may call this habit laziness, but it really is a form of learned helplessness. After some time, this person will no longer believe they can answer their own questions or perform the necessary actions to solve their own problems and instead they rely on others to do it for them. It is such a small habit, but one that can exponentially grow if fed.

Parents, teachers, Google, and bosses do this every day. Instead of opening up a dialogue or asking questions to really make that person think about the solution, they simply answer the question or solve the problem right off the bat.

How does this affect our health and life goals? We start *believing* we can't reach them. We start thinking that without help, accomplishing these goals is impossible. Without someone holding our hand every step of the way, they can't be done.

I can't stress this enough, this is a **_learned behavior_**.

How have you become successful at anything that you have done? How did you become a good tennis player? Or a good accountant? Anything.

Did someone sit down with you and tell you step-by-step exactly what move to make? Did they hold your hand and do it for you until you could take over? No. You learn by doing. You practice.

Now maybe along the way you met a better player or accountant who showed you some tips and tricks. Then you used those in your own strategic ways to develop your game or career. Maybe you got stuck on a specific issue and had to do some research to find out where you were making a mistake. You may have watched tennis players on television or read books about accounting to become even better and learn from the best in the game.

What is the common thread between all of these things?

You did them, no one else.

In these scenarios, you took the initiative to become good at your job or your hobby. This helped you become **worth more**. This is what made you successful. For those of you who have not been successful with your health and life goals, let me ask you, when you hit a roadblock did you take the initiative?

Did you do hours upon hours of research, trying to solve your problem?

Can you honestly say that you did absolutely everything in your power to get over that hurdle?

I already know the answer: it is __no__ or else you would have succeeded.

Before excuses come out or I hear something like, "But you don't understand," let me explain something: you're an incredible, capable person.

Memorize this quote by Marianne Williamson, "Our deepest fear is not that we are inadequate. Our deepest fear is that we are powerful beyond measure." <u>This is you</u>! You have all of the tools.

You have an incredible body that can move in infinite ways. You

have a mind that can conquer any problem if you try hard enough.

You have a willpower which is beyond that of any measurement.

There is absolutely no one else in this world who is going to be

better at your life, than you. <u>No one</u>. You simply have to take

action.

Key Takeaways:

- **Step away from learned helplessness by practicing your healthy habits and know you have the power to create your own success with practice.**

- **No one will ever be better at your life, than you.**

2.8: Turning Learned Helplessness into Self-Efficacy

I was guilty of learned helplessness myself for so long. The Millennial way: Google *EVERYTHING!*

At my first job I luckily had a wonderful boss and mentor. He challenged me with every project and conversation. He would come to my desk with an open-ended question, "How should we construct this?"

Sometimes it was a puzzle or a riddle to break up the day.

We'd go back and forth on certain ideas and he would challenge my solutions, "But what if this popped up or that?" It was so foreign at the time and at first panic set in.

What the hell is he doing?

Is this a test?

I'm fucked, *soooo* fired after this.

Over time I understood his purpose was just to help get me away from learned helplessness. So often, freshly groomed college grads come into the work force needing to be spoon fed what to do. This is not an insult; it's a fact of how we grew up. With the technology we now have, every generation is guilty of learned helplessness.

However, by questioning me and really making me critically examine every solution, my mentor completely changed the way I thought.

I felt empowered!

Confident!

I knew I could get any solution I needed with some planning and critical thinking. I was more relaxed and I didn't try to rush into my answers anymore. I didn't rely on anyone else for the answers either. I took the calm and collected route. I was truly *believing in myself* and *my capabilities*.

When it comes to health and success, you are no different than any other person out there. *You are a human*. You are part of a species of over *7 billion* other beings. If other people can be healthy, happy, and accomplish their goals, then so can you!

When many friends or clients approach me asking for advice, they usually expect some ground-breaking secret formula. When I suggest something as simple as eating more whole foods using the 80/20 rule, (which we will discuss later), or using positive thinking to change their perspective, they are hardly satisfied.

They still think there is some secret algorithm that I know and they don't. They can't accept that we are the same or that the solutions might take a little patience. Then they might say something that drives me absolutely crazy, "That's easy for you to say, you obviously have a better metabolism, better talents, better bone structure, have more time, less responsibilities."

You name it, they will try to create a reason why I am better than them or why I can do more. They look for an excuse. *A scapegoat.* They see my body or lifestyle and assume. And you know what they say when you assume? You make an **ass** out of **you** and **me**.

Most people don't want to accept the fact that I am healthier than them because I have researched scientific studies for hours, every single day, for the last seven years to learn about health from every angle, and then I acted on that research. <u>They don't see that I practice what I preach in this book every single day without fail because I have created successful habits.</u>

They don't see that I have struggled in the past immensely to get here. I couldn't do a single pullup when I first started working out, and I was lifting 10 pound dumbbells. Every week for half a decade I practiced trial-and-error with nutritional habits.

They didn't see my day-to-day habits. They weren't in my home to see me constantly reading, researching, and growing for <u>years</u>, changing my lifestyle and frame of mind to be conducive to my goals.

Like I said when we first started this book: *I am not a special butterfly.*

I simply instilled good habits, stepped away from learned helplessness, and believed in myself and my abilities.

Almost every person who has ever been great did not wondrously achieve this overnight. There are a few outliers who were handed down fortunes or have amazing genetics. These are outliers. Savants. We are talking about .0001% of the population.

What have the rest of successful people done? *Worked day in and day out.* There is no guaranteed predisposition to success or health. The 10,000-hour rule is hotly debated, but history has shown us that in most cases it is true. Football players are athletic, but there are a ton of athletic guys out there. Why did some make it to the NFL and some didn't?

Hard work.

They trained.

They made no excuses.

They create a mindset that **they would not fail**.

They believed in themselves and knew they would succeed.

Then they trained some more.

No one held their hand step by step. No one did it for them. They achieved this success by believing in themselves, then proving it. We need to switch the habit of learned helplessness around and begin practicing what psychologist Albert Bandura defined as self-efficacy.

Self-efficacy is believing in your own ability. Not thinking or wanting, but <u>knowing</u> that you will accomplish your goals. It's never doubting your mind or yourself. Take think, should, would, could, probably, maybe, and any word like it, out of your vocabulary.

It's not, "I want to be healthy and get the girl or guy of my dreams."

It is, "***I am*** becoming the best version of myself through my health and ***I will*** get the girl or guy of my dreams."

Don't be creepy about it, but you get the point.

If you believe in yourself, then **you will be the most powerful person possible**. You can have control over your life, if you believe you do. In the words of Henry Ford, "Whether you think you can, or you think you can't, you're right".

Decide today that you're going to create the mindset that *will* make your dreams a reality and never look back. You *will* accomplish anything in life as long as you believe in yourself and take action.

Step away from learned helplessness, take responsibility of your destiny, and believe in yourself through self-efficacy. This confidence will create a wave of impact through every portion of your life.

Key Takeaway:

- **Self-efficacy is believing in your own ability; not thinking or wanting, but knowing you will accomplish your goals. Practice self-efficacy by believing in yourself and your capabilities, then get to work and prove it by accomplishing your goals.**

2.9: Superficial Problems Taking Over Our Time

Body Image….. oh body image, how you've crept into our lives via social media and destroyed us from the inside out. I didn't want to discuss this issue, but with its rise in attention lately, I feel I must.

Body image, body shaming, fat shaming, loving yourself for you who are, etc. Are all a waste of time. That's right, fat shaming is just as bad as loving yourself for who you are, and vice versa. Time spent sulking, hating, bragging, or being content, is all *wasted time* that could have been spent on self-improvement or something productive.

This is a completely **made up** fad that is subjective and different for every single person. Don't fall into this time-wasting trap!

I don't care if you're Arnold Schwarzenegger or a fat person who loves your body, self-improvement should **always** be a goal.

Do you know why Arnold Schwarzenegger is as successful as he is, in many facets of his life? Because he always strives for more. He doesn't sit around saying, "Wow, I'm so amazing, I love myself so much that I'm done improving." No, he went for the next title and the title after that. Then he went after his other goals. He didn't waste his time being vain and constantly thinking or worrying about himself or what others think.

Stop wasting your time.

If you consume yourself with accomplishing your goals, you won't have time to sit around and care who thinks what about you or your body. Worrying about your body image is something so superficial and unimportant, but we are actually letting it impede many parts of our lives.

Shutting out social media is honestly one of the best things you can do for yourself. Unless you use it as a marketing or business tool, it is pretty much useless and typically causes more harm than good. As a society, we waste so much time looking at *other* people's lives or worrying what *they* think about ours. It is time to stop this. It's time to stop comparing ourselves with others to only sulk about what we don't have.

On the flip side, if you're an overweight person going online and telling others that they're perfect the way they are, they don't need to change anything, etc. You're wasting your time and theirs. Encouragement is good, complacency is <u>not</u>.

As we explained before, health is about your entire being which in turn affects those other parts of your life: wealth, happiness, and love. You should always be striving to improve all of these areas. I hate to break it to you, but being overweight is not healthy or going to help those other three pillars.

Every time you catch yourself looking in the mirror or at the scale and sulking, revert back to your goals! Stop consuming your time with frivolous, superficial material.

This isn't just about social media. It could be gossip magazines, reality television, or even slandering others in real life with friends.

All of this is detrimental. It's not only wasted time but it's also *pulling you away* from success. When consumed with one of these wastes of time, ask yourself, "What am I doing right now that is contributing to my goals or improving myself?" Nothing, so do something that does contribute to them.

I know it's hard. I've been there! These superficial items are like negativity in that they are **diseases**. They infect our mood, way of thinking, and even our actions. Being mindful of them and their effects is the first step. You need to keep a positive mindset and always surround yourself with the right people, places, things, and ideas for success.

Next, you have to continually imbed your habits and actions within your goals. Stop focusing on something so trivial as looks or what others think and keep focusing on your future. The physical looks will come as your health improves, I promise, but don't waste your time worrying about something so small or reverting your goals back to something so unimportant. Always be thinking about the big picture!

Key Takeaways:

- **Stop wasting your time with superficial items that do not matter or worrying about what others think.**

- **When feeling any of the negative emotions above, revert back to your goals and consume yourself with them and your future.**

Chapter 3: The Lifestyle That Will Set Up Your Success

Your actions and thoughts define who you are as a human. If you always think negatively, eventually, you will become a very negative person. To the same degree, if you always try to take the easy way out, you will become lazy in many other parts of your life.

The collection of your daily habits strung together, is what creates your lifestyle. This is why all of a sudden going on a diet or trying a new workout routine does not create long-term results for 99% of people. You can't just pretend for one hour of the day you are going to change everything about yourself, then go back to all of your unhealthy habits for the other 23 hours of the day.

If you are only positive for one hour of the day, then have negative thoughts throughout the other 23 hours, you will still be a negative person. **Majority rules**.

You have to create the habit of positivity if you want it to last. The same goes for our lifestyle. We must change our daily habits to reflect a healthy lifestyle throughout our entire day, *not just for 1 hour in the gym.*

Our lifestyles and daily actions determine who we are and how we act. If you're stressed, sleep deprived, and sedentary, it shouldn't be a surprise if your personality reflects traits of irritability, tiredness, and depression. All of these things go far beyond your health.

How can we expect to make as much money as possible, if we have trouble getting through a work day?

How can we expect our partners to pour their hearts out to us, if we can't provide that same level of love and energy back?

How can we expect happiness, when our mind is not in its' best state? **We can't.**

When your lifestyle habits affect your health, they really affect the entire fabric of your life. Achieving healthy lifestyle habits can drastically improve your life and lead you that much closer to accomplishing your goals. To do this, you must create lasting healthy habits that will one day become *intuitive* and *subconscious*.

In this section, we will cover all of the most influential habits that affect our lifestyle. We will dive deep to form habits that will:

Develop better sleep patterns.

Get rid of pain.

Create stress coping mechanisms.

Increase your activity levels.

Construct daily rituals.

And help you live a more naturally balanced life.

With these habits you will experience a renewed vigor and revitalized body which will not only make your life more enjoyable, but also put you on the path to making your dreams come true.

Key Takeaways:

- **Your lifestyle is all of your daily habits strung together and these habits determine who you are and how you act.**

- **When your lifestyle habits affect your health they also affect your wealth, happiness, and love.**

3.1: Do Sleep On It

Oh, the feeling of a good night's sleep. Fresh energy pulsating through the body with a warm sensation blanketing us like the Mediterranean in July. The cocoon of linens that snuggle us into oblivion. That very first morning stretch creates an inexplicable feeling, as if God is personally surging vitality through every mitochondrion in our existence.

I hope that I don't have to convince you how important sleep is. Sleep regulates every function of your mind and body. It is responsible for healthy brain function, hormone levels, recovery, and everything in-between.

There have been vast amounts of research done on sleep and it all comes back to one conclusion: **sleep is our lifeline**. If you're sleep deprived over a long period of time you're much more likely to have many diseases and illnesses.[15]

In the short-term, you will not function mentally or physically anywhere near your best, which will lead you further away from your goals. Sleep truly needs to be a priority in your life. No matter how busy your life is, sleep should <u>never</u> be sacrificed.

I see it happen all the time, clients sacrifice sleep for working more on a project or business, while it ultimately just lowers the quality of their work as each day passes. If this is your issue, then work on your time management, do not sacrifice your sleep. Two hours of extra sleep could potentially double your productivity the next day, so do yourself a favor and stop creating that tradeoff.

When it comes to sleep we should aim for at least 7 hours per night. Preferably 8 or more is ideal. We should also limit noise and light pollution near our sleeping quarters. Even a little light from a charging toothbrush or noise from a vibrating cell phone can disrupt our entire sleeping pattern for the night. Limit these distractions for sound sleep.

Look around your bedroom right now. Identify all of the noise and light pollution sources in your room that you can change and write them down.

1. _____

_____

2. _____

_____

3. _____

_____

4. _____

_____

5. _____

_____

You could place your phone on silent so no chimes or vibrations are heard through the night. Close the bathroom door when your toothbrush is charging to limit this light source. Facing your alarm clock towards the wall or turning it upside-down can make a big difference in the pollution. Identify any object that could be interfering with your sleep and create a solution for it.

Next, sleep in whatever position you're most comfortable with because at the end of the day, if you're comfortable, you will most likely sleep your best. Try to also breathe through your nose and diaphragm before going to bed. This will calm your central nervous system and get you ready for a restful night.

An hour or so before you go to sleep, try to limit electronic usage. Our brains associate the bright blue light that emits from screens with daylight and being awake. Our brains unwind best with dim, orange light before sleeping, which is associated with *sunset and fire*. These blue and orange colors are measured using the Kelvin Scale.

If you must go on your computer or be on your phone leading up to bed time, a great app I suggest you use is *f.lux*.

This app actually changes the kelvin color of your screen to emulate the natural sunrise and sunset patterns in your geographical area. During the daytime your screen will be brighter, with a slight blue tint at a higher kelvin measurement, which signals the brain that it is day time and to be alert. At nighttime, the kelvin will change to a dimmer, more orange glow, emulating sunset and telling your brain it is time to wind down.

This is an excellent example of a technological advancement that encourages natural health in our modern world. This subtle change will help your sleep quality immensely.

The best part? It is *free* to download!

Full disclosure, I would never suggest or endorse any product that I don't use every day myself. This has been a product in my life every day for the past three years which has created excellent results for myself, my clients, and my family. This app is also extremely popular among the tech industry and with celebrities.

We will talk about night time routines later in the lifestyle section, which will help our brain relax and get our bodies ready for a great night's sleep. If you frequently have trouble falling asleep at night, I strongly suggest incorporating meditation and breathing techniques into your nightly routine.

These will help your various nervous systems relax and work together, enabling you to peacefully melt to sleep. We will cover more of these stress-relieving practices in depth through chapter 3.3.

If you have trouble falling asleep it is essential you get sunlight during the day. When sunlight hits your eyes it signals your brain to produce melatonin: *the sleep hormone.*[51] Production of melatonin during the day also *increases* the production at night which helps you fall asleep much easier.[51] Without ample amounts of sunlight our bodies don't produce enough melatonin and our systems become out of sync. Something as simple as 15 minutes of sunlight during the day could make the difference between a great night's sleep and tossing and turning all night.

All of these solutions are **very simple** and **free**.

There is no reason not to try any or all of them out, especially if you're currently having trouble with your sleep. We should all strive for the best sleep quality possible every day and at least 7 hours per night.

It is helpful to create a designated time when you will go to sleep every work-day, no matter what! Planning it out, can make the difference between saying you will do something and actually doing it. In saying that, write down your work-day sleep schedule below:

Day of the Week: I Will Go to Sleep at: I Will Wake Up at:

_____   _____   _____

_____   _____   _____

_____   _____   _____

_____   _____   _____

_____   _____   _____

_____   _____   _____

I am not a Nazi, so only plan out the days you work, as these are naturally the days that you will have to be more structured.

Make a routine that you go to bed at a certain time every night with no exceptions during the work week. This really is one of those healthy habits that is a no brainer. A good night's rest could ultimately be the difference maker between us <u>accomplishing our goals</u> or *falling just short*.

Key Takeaways:

- **Your sleep quality affects your health, mood, and productivity.**

- **Limit light and noise pollution around your sleeping quarters.**

- **If you have trouble falling asleep incorporate f.lux, sunlight, and meditation into your lifestyle.**

- **Create consistency with your sleep habits.**

3.2: Relieving Pain the Old Fashion Way

Pain treatment in America is a gigantic industry that makes hundreds of billions of dollars every year.

Notice I said *treating*, not curing.

That is because, this is what most Western medicines do, treat, cover up, mask, suppress: most never get to the *root* of the problem.

I respect Western medicine as there are certain treatments and surgeries that are incredibly innovative and helpful. However, much of medicine in America is treated as a business. Without continual problems those businesses are hurt by falling profits. This is why a constant theme in our culture is to use treatments that lead to a perpetuation of the underlying problem so that profits can continually be made.

Why change our frame of mind and meditate to relieve stress, when we can take anxiety medication or anti-depressants?

Why change our motor patterns and posture, when we can alleviate joint pain with a pain pill every single day?

Why eat good food, when we can simply take a cocktail of pills to suppress our indigestion, heartburn, cholesterol, and blood pressure?

We create a cycle of dependency on these medications. This is why when almost every person goes on blood pressure or cholesterol medication, they stay on them for the rest of their lives. This dependency is just another form of learned helplessness adding to our problems.

We don't take responsibility: we just want the quick fix. We are then somehow *shocked* when a doctor comes into the room and announces we have **cancer**, **heart disease**, or any other **serious ailment**.

Everything I lay out in this book can help with pain to a degree. The psychological principles above will help ease much of our social, mental, and emotional pain. The nutritional habits and principles in the next section will help with internal pains and serve as a kind of internal medicine.

For right now, I want to talk about using one easy solution to cure much of our physical pain. This would be our lower back pain, cervical back pain, shoulder pain, neck pain, hip pain, knee pain, and even ankle pain.

It is important to repeat that 80% of Americans will suffer low back pain sometime in their life.[7] This is just lower back pain. We aren't even covering all of the other joints, ligaments or muscles in the body that are frequently injured. Physical therapy clinics are alive and well because of how injured our society is. Physical therapists do an amazing job at rehabilitating patients, but what if we could avoid the majority of those visits to begin with?

Being pain-free is an important detail in accomplishing our goals. If we are in pain, we will be constantly distracted. We won't be able to work as hard for as long. Pain affects us emotionally and mentally as much as it does physically. Our relationships, goals, success, and happiness will all suffer if we are in pain. When it comes to our physical pain we must develop a better understanding of our bodies.

You see everything in our body is connected.

Everything!

The movement of our ankles, affects the movement of our knees, which affects our hips, which affects our lower back, and so on.

The body is a *kinetic chain*, constantly dispersing energy and force throughout itself. The solution to our physical pain is not talked about much past our early childhood. Our mothers would tell us not to slouch when we were 6, but now that we are adults, we are inadvertently forced to everyday.

What lifestyle habit severely affects our physical pain? **Posture and our body mechanics**. America has become a breeding ground for bad posture. Look at our social norms:

We stick children in desks for hours a day once they turn 5.

We stick adults in cubicles for 8 hours per day for years on end.

We create vehicles that encourage bad posture for hours of driving.

We sit on nice cushy couches which completely annihilate our spines.

To understand how our posture has become so bad, we first must understand our natural kinesiology.

Naturally, we are not meant to sit in chairs. We are not meant to lounge on super soft, cushy surfaces for hours on end. I can't stress this enough. These are physiological proven facts through *evolution* and the *human body* itself.

We are designed with motor patterns perfectly programmed into our central nervous system. From birth we are programmed to move a certain way. Our bodies naturally want to take the path of least resistance and use good body mechanics.

For example, what is the natural resting position for the human body? No, not sitting.

It is actually the deep squat.[16]

That is a flat foot, ass a couple of inches off the ground, ankles in a 45-degree dorsiflexion, knees over toes, squat. This is how we were physically designed to rest, shit, and perform any given task from cooking to picking up things off the ground.

In the Western world, our posture has become so poor that most of us can't even get in to this position to begin with, *let alone rest there.*

Look at any child. They do not learn to deep squat, they do it naturally from the moment they can place pressure on their two feet. Ask a young child to pick up an object and they will squat to do so. They won't bend over with straight legs.

They will deep squat.

This is a natural movement pattern engrained in our biology. The only reason this motor pattern has changed is because we strip it away from our children as soon as they go off to school or as Coach Shane Trotter calls them: bad habit factories.[43]

It is not just our resting position that we get wrong, it's also the way we stand, walk, and move. Most Americans walk with their shoulders' and neck's forward, ass back behind them like Donald Duck and with a large curve in their lower back, all while slamming down heel first. This is **not** how we were meant to walk.

Our gait (walking stride), has been destroyed through years of bad postural habits and the use of shoes. Our feet are weak, our ankles are unstable, and we have absorbed a vast amount of tension over time which is literally changing the structure of our bodies.

The evidence is astounding that posture is most likely the most major cause of back and shoulder pain in the Western world.[18] Here's the deal. We, in America, have astounding rates of back and shoulder pain. Look at tribal cultures that practice good resting and standing posture, and you will see that back and shoulder pain is almost **non-existent**.[18]

This is not a coincidence.

While our cultures are vastly different, the common thread we share is the ability to rest and move. That is the one attribute in all of our cultures that we approach so differently. After comparing our sedentary, pain-ridden, poor posture lifestyle, to their active, pain-free, perfect posture lifestyle, I don't think it takes a rocket scientist to figure out that our postural habits might be creating our physical pain.

We are meant to walk with a neutral pelvis, with a spine that is a *J shape* rather than an S shape, with our butt muscles constantly activated to continually supporting our weight, and with our belly buttons drawn inward for a nice, tall posture.[18]

Our necks should be in line with the rest of our back, which should be pretty straight besides the last few vertebrae and our tail bone. Our shoulders should be pinned back, with our chest outward.

Lastly, we are actually meant to land on our mid and fore foot, not our heel. If you don't believe me, walk barefoot for a day landing heel first, then come back and let me know how much pain you're in by the end of the day. I'd be willing to bet it will take a couple of weeks for those heel bruises to rehabilitate.

The only reason we are able to walk on our heels now is because the cushion of our shoes enables us to. Which brings me to my next point, *shoes aren't natural*.

Our shoes act as casts, paralyzing our feet muscles and eventually making them so weak, they don't even function right. About 20% of our bodies' bones and muscles are contained in our feet, this is how important they truly are. Almost every action we take stems from our feet. They are our lifeline for movement.

Utilizing our bare feet and proper posture as much as possible, can drastically reduce our physical pain and bring our joints back to normal health. I often hear excuses like, "But my feet are flat, I need shoes."

Your flat feet don't need shoes. *Your shitty shoes created your flat feet*! Your feet are flat because the muscles in your arches are **weak**. By giving your feet even more support you are making them even *weaker*. Your feet have to rely more and more on cushion to be able to support themselves until they can no longer support themselves without said cushion.

Another vicious cycle of learned helplessness.

Your feet, ankles, knees, hips, and backs will only get stronger by having to support themselves from the ground up. Without challenging our feet, they and the rest of our bodies will remain weak and vulnerable to serious injury.

Ok, ok, we get it!

We aren't living the way our bodies were meant too!

But this is the modern world!

What are we supposed to do, throw out all of our shoes and quit our jobs? No, of course not. As with all of our solutions, we are going to create small changes that will ripple throughout our day and create good health benefits long-term.

Our first small change is going to come in the form of **balance**. Try to create balance in your life between being barefoot and wearing shoes. If you wear shoes for 8 hours a day at your job, try to spend a majority of the rest of your day barefoot. Going barefoot will help reinforce a proper walking stride and posture.

You will be amazed at how great this will feel.

It is freeing!

Don't just go barefoot and sit on the couch for 8 hours either, go outside, go to a park! Even doing menial tasks like taking the trash out to the curb can be done while going barefoot. It is time to gain the strength back in our feet and ankles.

Another great way to make a difference is to wear minimalist shoes when you do have to wear shoes. These are shoes with minimal padding in the soles. Minimalist and barefoot shoe brands are popping up everywhere and most of them are not anywhere near as ugly as Vibram Fivefingers. There are stylish tennis shoes, flats, and dress shoes now made by minimalist brands you can wear during any part of your day.

When it comes to posture we need to correct ourselves. You need to reverse your bad habits and practice perfect posture **as much as possible**. This should be done throughout your entire day, <u>every single day</u>. It really doesn't take much effort to be mindful of your posture.

In order to be able to self-correct yourself, you need to first actually feel what perfect posture is. It is not enough just to read this, you have to be able to feel the position and memorize it through a motor pattern.

So stand up right now, please!

Go to a wall that doesn't have any stylish furniture or cute family pictures on it. Now stand with your back against the wall.

Your heels, butt, shoulder blades, and head should all be touching the wall. Whenever in standing posture try to be as tall as possible with your shoulders back and down.

A great cue for standing posture is to push your heels into each other and clench your butt. Try it right now, squeeze that booty like you're crushing the juiciest peach that has ever been picked.

This will help level out your pelvis and create a smaller lordotic curve in your back. Through constant practice it will also create a firm booty that you can be proud of. By doing this simple cue you're creating more support for your body by utilizing your most powerful muscle.

You should not have a very large space between the wall and your lower back, if you do, push your hips forward slightly to straighten your spine.

Next, draw in your belly button just a little bit and create a supportive core by bracing. Finally, after you're done with this sentence, look forward and take a few moments to feel this posture out and *memorize this body positioning.*

Below, write down which areas you need to work on the most. Did you have to actively push your head back towards the wall because it was used to being forward?

Before squeezing your heels together was there a very large curve in your lower back that became much smaller after doing so?

Were your shoulders slumped forward and did you have to consciously pin them back?

Did your heels not touch the wall at first?

Did drawing in your belly button make you instantly taller?

Now that you know what perfect posture feels like, write down three areas of your posture that you need to continually focus on.

1. _____

_____

2. _____

_____

3. _____

_____

You can even grab a friend or family member and examine each other's posture to see where the weak links are. It can't be stressed enough how important posture is at all times of the day.

A common complaint I hear from many people is that they have back pain after doing household chores like laundry, the dishes, or vacuuming. Even when we perform small tasks such as folding clothes or doing the dishes, we usually have terrible posture. We bend over at the waist with straight legs which puts a huge strain on our lower backs.

Think of what this does to your back when you do these tasks every single day for years. Over time it is no wonder that you have lower back pain. You can fix this with good postural cues and changes.

The easy solution when folding clothes or washing the dishes, is to start out in a perfect, tall, standing posture. Next push your knees forward into the cabinet in front of you while also pushing your hips back, like in the deadlift position.

From here do the dishes or laundry in the hip hinge position with your hips pushed back, a neutral spine, and your shoulders slightly back. Now we are utilizing better posture and body mechanics. We are using our hips as the weight bearer instead of our backs and this will put way less stress on your lower back and lead to decreased pain over time.

Another complaint I often hear is having back pain after vacuuming. When most people vacuum they are leaning forward, hunched over, with a curved back in a flexed position. Again, this creates huge strain on the lower back. Having good posture with the shoulders back, standing tall, drawing in the belly button, and flexing the butt muscles will fix this body mechanic and your lower back pain. Incorporate good postural mechanics into every movement you do. The key is to always be mindful of your body. Have you ever heard of a friend or coworker who is **big** and **strong**, but threw their back out by picking up something <u>small</u> like a *toy or shoe*?

I have heard this countless times and it is because while these big guys might practice good postural habits while lifting weights, this usually disappears once they step foot outside of the gym. Most of us go throughout our day without ever realizing what our bad habits are. Take some time to examine your postural habits and see where you're making mistakes. From here practice perfect standing and moving posture, while also substituting deep squatting for sitting, as much as possible. This is very easy; you just need to make it a habit.

I know this may seem weird. I know this is counter-culture for us Americans, but this is so crucial. This deep squat position is so important for the health of our hips, spine, and overall mobility.

Deep squat instead of sitting when you play with a pet. Take deep squatting breaks while you watch television or read. Try to increase your time each instance that you deep squat.

Doing this even **5 *minutes*** a day will create lasting impacts in your joint health and mobility. You can make it part of your morning and nightly routine by doing it for just two minutes on each end of the day.

If you can't get into the full position, work into it with practice by holding on to a support while you get used to the deep squat. The key to all of our postural positions is to use the hips not the back. It really doesn't take much effort to be mindful of your posture. You now have the tools to eliminate your pain, so why not use them?

There is no excuse.

You can make the effort to be conscious of your posture or ***spend tens of thousands of dollars*** over the course of your life on pain pills, doctors' appointments, and God forbid, surgeries to temporarily relieve your pain symptoms which will always come back. Think of all the things you could do with tens of thousands of dollars, wow. I think the first option sounds a little better.

You will also be surprised at the way people perceive you. A perfect posture is a *strong* posture. It is a gladiator firmly holding his position upon an army of beasts. It will change the way coworkers, family, friends, and even members of the same or opposite sex that you're trying to attract, view you. You will seem just that:

Strong.

Confident.

In control.

Don't be surprised if you pick up more clients, create new friendships, and attract more people in general. There is a huge psychology to the way people view you physically and posture is usually one of the first things others notice.

There is also a great degree of psychology involved in the way we view ourselves. Bad posture is associated with inner thoughts of insecurities and uncertainty. While perfect posture is associated with an internal thought process that is *confident and ready.*[19]

How you see yourself is often how others view you. You can't expect others to view you as attractive, want to do business with you or think you are capable of success, if you don't **first feel** these attributes about yourself.

When talking about posture, we should be mindful of our center of gravity. Our center of gravity will determine where and how much stress is placed on our joints. We always want to be evenly distributed with our weight and in the most advantageous position as possible. The same is true when carrying an object. We never want to let the object move us.

An example, would be carrying a box and letting the weight of the box momentously carry us forward. This is a recipe for disaster. By changing our body mechanics so that our hips are pushed forward and we are slightly leaning back, the weight will now be evenly distributed throughout our body and we can confidently handle the box.

If we are smart about how we distribute our weight, our body positioning, and our posture we can naturally eliminate most of the joint pain we commonly encounter in our daily lives. I can't stress this enough, *always use the hips*!

Lastly, let's address that **demon** in the corner of the room, **the chair**.

Just look at it....

Arrogant and cocky, yet it draws us to it like a **black hole** engulfing stars one by one until an entire galaxy is struck from the sky. If it were up to me, all chairs would be burned, I tell you, burned!!!

Maybe not all, but you can guess how much I loathe these modern torture devices. However, to their relief, I do not decide the fate of all of the chairs in the world, so let's explore some practical solutions that will help create a healthy lifestyle while still letting these monstrosities exist.

Since we spend the majority of our day at work, the easiest solution to sitting less is to ask for a standing desk at work. These are becoming more and more common as vast amounts of research are starting to equate sitting as the new smoking,[20] and an important predictor for chronic disease risk.[21]

If you use one of our previous principles to explain to your human resources director how beneficial it is to invest in employees, there is a good chance they will make the right choice and invest in you as an employee with a standing desk. There is recent research showing that standing desks *increased* workers' productivity by **45%**.[50]

Forty-five percent!

That would be accomplishing **900 extra hours** of work every year, without ever working an extra hour. No human resources director can dispute those kinds of results. When in doubt, start citing research articles including the ones in this book. Explain this isn't a luxury, but a necessity for health purposes.

Whether you have a standing desk or not, it is always important to maintain good posture. If we have a standing desk but we are still slouching with rounded shoulders and a forward neck, our bodies will still not be happy with us.

With a standing desk it is comfortable to transition between sitting and standing frequently. In saying this, the same applies to sitting. When sitting it is important to still maintain a good posture with your shoulders back, neck in line with the rest of your spine, and feet flat on the floor.

It is easy to fall victim to bad postural habits when we return to our cozy homes after a long day. Don't let this be the case. A little mindfulness in your posture and body mechanics will go a long way to securing a pain-free future.

Aren't you tired of living in pain?

Are you ready to <u>fix</u> that and <u>prevent future pain</u> from occurring?

Then it is time to correct your posture and practice these good habits as often as possible. It doesn't matter if you're currently a fit gym attendee or a couch potato, bad backs have a way of catching up to every American who doesn't regularly practice perfect posture. Do *yourself and your future-self* a favor and make this habit a staple in your lifestyle to correct and avoid pain.

Key Takeaways:

- **Always practice perfect posture and incorporate deep squatting throughout your day in small intervals.**

- **Be aware of your body positioning during every activity from lifting heavy objects to performing household chores, and always evenly distribute your body weight and position.**

- **Utilize a standing desk at work, balance being barefoot during the rest of your day, and avoid long periods of sedentary sitting.**

3.3: Crush Stress in Its' Tracks

It should come to no surprise how detrimental immense stress is in our lives. Stress has a way of trickling down and affecting much more than the initial item we were stressing about. Have you ever blown up at someone or over something, that was incredibly stupid? Of course you have, we all have! A food item is spoiled and we are mad at the universe.

Damn you milk!

Damn you to Hell!

Our significant other does something that we don't like and it spirals in to a huge fight. The catalyst of many of our blow ups is usually *stress* that eventually boils over.

I know this is counter-culture in the United States, but the research does not lie, nor do the millions of testimonials of successful people who have made this action a daily habit. I am talking about meditation.

Before you shut this out or think it is only for Tibetan monks who piss off the edge of Everest, hear me out. Meditation is so powerful it has been shown to actually change the structure of the brain in as little as eight weeks.[25] Meditation can help you clear your mind and remove all of the tension throughout your body. Meditation is also not hard to do. In fact, it is *almost impossible* to mess up.

The simplest form of meditation is taking deep diaphragmatic breaths and focusing on your breathing. Diaphragmatic breathing is simply breathing through your diaphragm or belly, rather than your chest.

Chest breathing signals **panic** in your brain and reverts your body to fight or flight instincts. Diaphragmatic breaths signal *calm and relaxation: a resting state.*[26]

Some of us may go an entire day without a single good diaphragmatic breath, which leaves us in a constant state of stress whether we realize it or not. Throughout your day stop every once in a while and examine your breathing.

Being mindful of your breath is very important and easy to do. You can take deep breaths while at your desk or while doing household chores. Doing this throughout your day can drastically reduce your stress without you even realizing it. You just have to remember to do it and create the habit. Eventually, diaphragmatic breathing will become automatic.

For meditation purposes, we can start out by simply performing deep breaths through our diaphragms. An easy queue to help breathe diaphragmatically, is to breathe into the back of your throat. This will force deep breaths into our stomach, instead of our chest.

Try it right now!

Lay on the floor, on your back with your knees bent. When you inhale, breathe through the back of your throat and into your stomach or diaphragm. With every inhalation your stomach should raise upwards, with every exhalation your stomach with empty and flatten down again. Try varying your breath holds.

Do some **short powerful** breaths and couple this with *deep drawn* in breaths, all while clearing your mind and tension. Simply do this for 5 to 10 minutes whenever you're feeling stressed out or overwhelmed.

You can do sessions where you solely use deep, long-held breaths to calm your body. You can use forceful inhalation and exhalation to excite your various nervous systems and culminate an adrenaline response. Use breath counts to synchronize your breathing, count in five seconds, hold for five seconds, and exhale out for five seconds. Do the same pattern, but with one second counts. Try all of these drills and the effects will be *dramatic*.

You can do short, forceful breaths in the morning to awaken your nervous system and hormones. Work on long, relaxing breaths at night to create a calming effect over the entire body as if you were bathing in chamomile.

There are tons of meditation tracks on YouTube that will help your mind relax and get rid of the extreme silence which can be distracting. You can use any slow, calming song you enjoy. I personally use theta, alpha, and delta wave tracks from YouTube and vary them depending on my mood or what I want to accomplish with that meditation session.

Experiment and find what works *best for you*!

From here you can progress into more advanced techniques of meditation varying from focusing on a state of emotion, an object, or even a goal. There is research that actually shows meditation can protect the brain against dementia and Alzheimer's disease.[27] Multiple studies have now shown that meditation used by monks and nuns can actually **slow brain aging**, which decreases the occurrence and severity of the diseases above.[27]

This is incredible! This is big picture stuff!

We are no longer talking about stress relief for a day, we are talking about actual *longevity* and *terminal disease prevention*.

With the overwhelming increase in dementia and Alzheimer's disease rates in America, this is huge news.

Now there are other ways to reduce stress. Maybe you like kickboxing after a hard workday, reading a few pages of a fantasy novel or watching your favorite television show to reduce your stress. Those are fine methods too, but they will not give us the same **cognitive** benefits as the meditation and breathing drills. When doing the drills above, you are solely focusing on your relaxation and breathing. **There are no other distractions**.

You are not preoccupying your mind with some other task or diverting your attention from the tension in your body. You are focusing directly on your mental state which will help you clear your mind and tension much easier and more effectively. Use small meditation breaks during your work day.

Get out and meditate at a park to listen to the calming sounds of nature around you.

Include this in your morning and nightly routines.

This could help you break through a plateau at work, help you brainstorm a new idea by rejuvenating your mind, or simply help you avoid a stressful blow up.

Set some time aside for yourself and use these life-altering practices. You can involve a friend, significant other or even make it a family affair. Invest in yourself, your health, and your brain by making this a staple of your lifestyle.

Key Takeaways:

- **Practice diaphragmatic breathing for stress relief throughout the day.**

- **Use meditation practices for longevity, terminal disease prevention, and to create a better you.**

3.4: Move Baby, Move

In many meta-analyses, there is a very common thread between all of the healthiest cultures: they walk a lot. We are endurance creatures by biology. Our energy systems and bodies are built for the long haul. We are well designed to move for long periods of time at a gentle pace.

Office work and a sedentary lifestyle throws this off.

We are **not** designed for a sedentary life. This is why so many health consequences pop up when we live without much movement. A constant theme I want to instill in our lifestyles is to <u>move more often</u>.

Simple. Move more. Instead of not moving, do the opposite and move.

Like we noted in the introduction, the average American sits for 13 hours a day. Combine this with the amount of time we sleep and we are almost never moving anymore! We drive everywhere. When we park, we try to get the closest parking spot possible. We take elevators over the stairs even when are traveling to the second floor.

Come on! What does all of this really come down to? Some may say convenience, but in reality, it is due to laziness. We intentionally try to move as least as possible. This mindset eventually creeps in and prevents us from exercising even small amounts. Laziness is like a drug. Netflixing that next episode on the couch is taking a hit.

Mmm yea, wasn't that hit nice, how about another? Then we wind up watching more and more episodes until several bags of snacks lay desolate on the floor and sugar plums are dancing in our heads. Eventually, this becomes a habit and we crave the *laziest solutions possible* throughout our entire life.

You become lazy at work.

You try to take shortcuts with your learning and growth.

You prioritize mindless entertainment over your goals and loved ones.

When you perpetuate laziness it isn't just your health that suffers, all of your goals and those pillars of life are pushed back as well.

First, with every issue discussed thus far we have addressed what the problem was. Now to change it, we go back to our central theme of *balance*. You don't need to make every minute of your day about moving and staying active, but you do need to keep in mind how sedentary you are and how much this negatively affects your life in so many different ways. You know you need to make a change, but you are not sure where to start.

When making these changes you always want to start out small. One of the best ways to start off a day and wake up your central nervous system, is with a simple five-minute walk. Another great, small implementation is taking frequent breaks at work to move.

Regardless of the desk you have at work, you should incorporate movement into your entire day for a healthy lifestyle.

You can do this by moving more frequently with small breaks or by physically moving your muscles even when we are sedentary. To start with the latter, moving these muscles is as easy as contracting them. This is better known to the *bros* of the world as *flexing*.

Muscle contraction is a powerful thing. It gets your blood flowing, releases endorphins, and feels incredible![22] Animals do full body muscle contractions every time they get up to move. You know when you first wake up and go into a deep stretch, arching your back and flexing your legs straight as hard as you can in bed; it feels like God is personally pumping steroids through those denim monsters.

Well, it feels the same way after being sedentary for hours. Contract your muscles while sitting, standing, or get up and do it on a break. Hold every contraction for at least five seconds. Do it with every muscle from head to toe. Here is my personal routine I use on my breaks.

Go on your tip toes to flex your calves.

Straighten your legs as hard as you can and target those quads.

Clench your gluteus maximus like you're protecting your booty in the prison showers!

Contract your core like you're getting ready for a punch.

Extend your arms downward and back to flex your triceps.

From here, go straight into a bicep and upper back squeeze.

Once you're done there, bring your arms across your chest to target the ol' pecs.

Finally open your jaw as wide as possible to contract your neck muscles.

This might sound weird, but *it feels incredible.*

DO IT! DO IT RIGHT NOW!

Do this a couple times a day at work and you will feel like a new person after sitting or standing for a while. Let's couple this with physically moving our bodies for an even better balance.

Now in the corporate world or work force, we can't be strolling around the hallways or job site all day. However, taking breaks every 30 minutes to get a little movement in and walk around is not unrealistic. In fact, if you do take these breaks it is proven you will be more focused and recharged when you do get back to work.[23,24] If your boss makes a comment about your movement, back it up with your work.

Explain to him or her that it helps your productivity, then **prove it**.

There is no argument why you can't take breaks and support your health when you're performing at your highest. This movement is a form of investing in yourself. Those three minute breaks you take every half hour will produce a <u>huge</u> outcome in your work. The mind does not do well in a constant grind. Like talked about in the previous section, you have to balance the yin with the yang.

It is helpful to have a ***little getaway*** at work. Somewhere desolate, where you can go to relax or get in a few movements throughout the day.

At my first job, it was a gym that I knew was empty every day from 9:00 to 11:30. I would go in there to lie on a mat and close my eyes for a couple minutes or to do a few stretches and exercises. At my last job in the corporate world it was an empty stairwell and a park across the street. I would use the stairwell to do push-ups or stretches, like deep lunges up the stairs. The park was my getaway at lunch and during extended breaks to get some sunshine and relax.

Find your getaway, it could be an empty conference room that is rarely used or a grassy median at the back of the parking lot, but this small slice of paradise will help you unwind and provide a few moments of **Zen** through the course of your work day.

Back to movement.

This is not something that I can create a manual for. I don't know you, your current schedule or your lifestyle. You have to take personal responsibility for your own lifestyle and movement. This isn't something to stress or constantly track. You just need to create the habit through *regular practice*.

Gradually ramp up your activity levels every week or so by adding in a few extra minutes of movement throughout your day to create a more active lifestyle over time. Think of three small ways you can add in slightly more movement throughout your day.

1. _____

_____

2. _____

_____

3. _____

_____

While Fitbits and other fitness walking trackers are great for the sedentary American lifestyle, you also want a wide variety of movements. It is good for your joints to hang, climb, jump, crawl, and perform every other movement your body is capable of. Not only is it important from a physical perspective, but physical activities create <u>neuroplasticity</u> in the brain: *which is the brains ability to adapt and create new neural pathways.*

Dancers are famous for frequently displaying high levels of neuroplasticity because they are constantly learning new movements and routines.[28] The brain has to adapt to acquire and develop expertise in new movements; thus, you should always be challenging your brain with a variety of movements to keep sharp.

It is also fun to challenge your body. Walking in a straight path can even put a hyperactive child who just devoured an entire package of Skittles to sleep. Balance on a curb, jump over a small gravel bed, dance your heart out, hang from a tree, the possibilities are **endless**. If you make movement <u>*fun*</u>, you will not only think of your breaks as necessities, but you will <u>*crave them*</u>.

Key Takeaways:

- **Keeping active throughout the day is more important than an hour in the gym, avoid a sedentary lifestyle like the plague.**

- **Vary your movements, take small breaks frequently at work, use the muscle contracting techniques above, and find your little getaway to improve yourself and your productivity.**

3.5: Morning and Nightly Rituals

What is a common trait of many of the most successful people on this planet? They have rituals. Not *Illuminati*, secret society rituals. I am talking about habits they use to create routines to get them ready for everything in their day and routines that let them unwind at the end of the day, to get the rest needed at night. This is so *crucial*. Sometimes we don't truly grasp how <u>nonstop</u> and <u>stressful</u> our lives are until we take a step back and examine them.

Friends and family obligations.

Children and everything those little monsters bring.

Forty-hour plus work weeks.

Demanding jobs.

Financial stressors.

Constantly having errands to run from grocery store trips to car maintenance checks.

Everyday chores around the house.

We have more responsibilities now than ever before. This is why so many of these principles like investing in yourself are so important, because if you don't actively take steps to implement these strategies into your life then all of the **chaos** that regularly occurs will *wash them away.*

We have to make these strategies a focal point. We do this by understanding just how important they are. These rituals aren't just improving you in the moment, they are setting you up for *success throughout your entire life*. Preparing and planning are essential steps to anything in life. Without them, the chaos will **engulf** us.

These rituals should prepare you mentally, physically, and emotionally for the day. They also don't have to be very time intensive, 10-15 minutes on each side of the day will make a huge difference in your future success.

If you're an office worker this might mean doing active exercises like lunges, pushups, and hip circles to get your blood pumping and prepare for the sedentary hours ahead.

For a construction worker, it may mean stretching to become limber and ready for all of the stress the body will take on from eight hours of labor. For either person above, it may include meditation and breathing exercises to energize the mind for everything to come. On the other side of the day, it may be meditation to clear the mind and relax after a long day.

Maybe you enjoy a cup of tea every morning. Reading 10 pages to indulge in a fantasy novel. It could be looking at the morning news or enjoying a past time. Perhaps you and your significant other decide to give each other three minute massages.

Only you will be able to determine your routine. It should include a variety of activities that will encourage mental, physical, and emotional health throughout your life. After you have developed your morning and nightly rituals you simply have to make sure they happen.

Don't make excuses.

Always set aside the time at night and in the morning to make sure these happen. If that means waking up 15 minutes early, then **do it**. Set the alarm. These rituals will make a huge difference in your entire day and will help your mornings feel less rushed. They will let you recover better at night and sleep more soundly.

List out at least 3-5 healthy activities that you will string together to make a morning and nightly routine.

Morning Routine

1._____

2._____

3._____

4._____

5._____

Nightly Routine

1._____

2._____

3._____

4._____

5._____

If you do not ready your mind and body for the day, don't be surprised when chaos ensues and you become rundown, tired or overwhelmed. In sports, athletes don't come on to the field or court cold turkey without a warmup. That would be a recipe for disaster.

They also ice, get massages, and stretch after the game to make sure they are healthy and ready for the next game or practice to come. You may not be an athlete, but there is no difference. Your work is your sport. Their sport is their livelihood and your job is yours. If you want to perform accordingly, the same rules apply, so warm-up and cool down daily, champ!

Key Takeaways:

- **Develop a well-rounded routine that focuses on your mental, physical, and emotional health.**

- **Create consistency with your morning and nightly routines, always make time for them.**

3.6: Less Artificial, More Biological

How we have so forgotten our natural biology. Billboards, buildings, and street lights are so common place that it is hard to imagine what life was like without them. **Industrialization** is forged deeply into our contemporary world.

Most of the population is glued to the urban jungle and masses of steel, concrete, and rebar that *tower over them*. Few of us live a natural life in our modern times. What do I mean by living naturally? To answer that, we have to go back to the human animal.

We are an animal, remember? We forget how much our lives have changed in modern history, because the life we are living now is the only life we personally have ever known.

Let's go back to 99.99% of our time on this planet before desk jobs, fluorescent lighting, chairs, couches, and the endless dark matter of the internet. What did we do? We slept, hunted, foraged, traveled, moved in every way, and talked.

Nothing special. Nothing crazy. Just basic actions in life.

However, the basics were <u>everything</u>.

Some of these things may sound silly to focus on, but we have to realize how much our modern lives have reversed them in such a short amount of time. Before modern society, it would be pretty common to walk several miles every single day to hunt, look for new land, and forage food or useful items. We have now cut this down to walking the least amount of steps possible, moving only in linear ways, and strangling our feet in rubber and cloth.

We used to go to sleep a couple hours past sunset after spending a night around the fire talking to one another. We would then wake up with the sunrise. Nowadays, we go to sleep way too late after spending hours watching mindless television. We then wake up much earlier than sunrise in many cases.

We communicate more with friends and family, but ultimately, we talk less. Our communication is done through the artificial means of texting, emailing, and lists of emoji's. If you ever figure out what the hell a smiley faced cat, next to a pineapple, followed by an eggplant, with a beach, and a tennis racket actually means, please let me know! We spend less time than ever talking face to face. Which has effects much deeper than communication.

We have food cooked and prepared for us, rather than making it ourselves.

Lastly, we spend our days in artificially lit, fluorescent rooms, instead of outside with normal sunlight and Vitamin D.

Now don't leap to extremes. I am not suggesting we revert back to the caves and forests to live as our ancestors did. Nevertheless, it is always good to be aware of the historical ways that we naturally lived not so long ago.

With all things in this book and life you should always strive for some sort of *balance*. You can sleep better hours, closer to sunset and sunrise. You will cook more for yourself and cherish your relationship with the food you eat, all while developing your creative side. You need to incorporate small amounts of movement throughout your day, so that you are never completely stagnate for more than an hour. You should try to communicate more with the ones you love face to face and verbally, rather than through a screen. Finally, you desperately need more natural sunlight in your life.

This last point is *vital*.

There are so many diseases tied to Vitamin D deficiency. Depression, Parkinson's, Alzheimer's, low testosterone levels, and countless other health-related problems are <u>directly</u> correlated to Vitamin D deficiency.[29,30]

We were not meant to stay indoors all day. You need to start understanding that sunlight is important for **survival**, not just a tan. Even during cloudy days your skin soaks up the sun's rays. Sunlight is integral for your body and mind.

When you take small breaks at work, head outside for a few minutes instead of staying in the building. Take walks at lunch from time to time. Exercising and spending time outdoors with family and friends is another great way to get more sunshine. We don't have to go to the Great Plains. A neighborhood park with grass, trees, and a playground will do the trick. Think big!

Start ingraining time spent in the sun with your goals. It is obvious that sunlight has a lot to do with our mental health, which keeps your mind sharp and focused. This can relate to any goal in life.

Going outside for a break of fresh air and sunlight can instantly give you a new perspective and cognitively spark an innovative design or marketing platform. Your time outside could be the brainstorming environment your body craves! Make going outside a priority throughout your day, especially when you're stressed, overwhelmed, and need a break.

Small breaks and activities can easily add up to over an hour or two outside every day. This will create mental, emotional, and physical changes that will impact your goals and life.

Sunlight is crucially important for your eye health as well. If you stare at a computer screen all day *you need sunlight*! Our eyes need to be exposed to a <u>full spectrum</u> of light every day to maintain their health. No indoor lighting provides the same full spectrum of light as the sun does.

A fun exercise to do during a work break outside is to close your eyes and look towards the sun. Keep them closed, but continue to face towards the sun. You will feel the heat of the sun hitting your eye lids and you will see a lot of light even though your eyes are closed. After 30 seconds lower your head, look straight ahead and open your eyes. Your eyes will feel rejuvenated, colors will become more vibrant, and your mind will feel relaxed. Try this the next time your eyes feel tired and foggy at work.

Sunlight is important for healthy brain function which affects our nervous and hormonal systems.[52] Stepping outside for 5 minutes after you wake up in the morning to get a little sunlight in will help regulate your circadian rhythm, bring your body temperature back up to normal, and give you all of the cognitive benefits you desire to have a productive day.[52]

Want to build your business? *Get more sunlight*. Want to alleviate stress, become the best version of yourself and regain true happiness? **Get more sunlight**.

Strive to utilize more time of your day living a natural life. Our biology and history exist for a reason and there are *drastic* effects when we go against them. For instance, a research study by the University of Colorado showed that camping in nature for one week can actually reset our circadian clocks and hormonal levels.[36]

It is that simple, camping outside and being exposed to sunrise and sunset can get rid of insomnia, hormonal imbalances, and even depression.

Many of our modern problems can be cured with things right in front of our faces. Things that exist all around us and have been here for a really, really long time. Balancing a more natural life into your modern world can have fantastic results for your health and long-term success. Implement some of those small changes we talked about above and your happiness, wealth, health, and love will naturally flourish.

Key Takeaways:

- **Balance a more natural lifestyle to satisfy your biological needs.**

- **Incorporate regular bouts of sunlight exposure to increase your work productivity and for healthy eye, brain, and hormone function.**

- **Try the stress relieving eye exercise above for rejuvenated vision throughout the day!**

3.7: Puff, Puff

This is going to be very short.

However, I do have to put in a passage about cigarette smoking. Luckily, this is on the decline as we become more educated and progressive as a society. I am not going to cite any scientific information about why cigarette smoking is bad......because it is everywhere.

Turn on the radio, television, or read any daily news site and you will see countless information about the negative health effects from smoking cigarettes. This is a habit that must be stopped for a healthy lifestyle.

Whenever you are smoking ask yourself, "Is this helping me get closer to my goals? Is this helping my family? Is this helping me be the person I want to be?" The answer to all of these is an astounding NO.

Make it personal as with your other habits and create some accountability. Be mindful of your smoking. Does it taste good? How does your mouth feel?

Put pressure on yourself to do the right thing. Whenever you are about to smoke simply ask, "Do I need this? Why am I doing this? Is there something else I could do instead to relive my stress like breathing exercises?" Sometimes slowing things down and logically looking at the situation will help you get away from the automatic habit.

If you have an oral or hand fixation, carry a squeeze ball or a food item to chew on that will relieve this fixation rather than relying on a cigarette.

There are plenty of ways to stop smoking. Make it personal. Be accountable. And take action to stop this terrible habit for good.

Key Takeaways:

- **Use any other stress relieving method besides smoking.**

- **Think of your goals and your loved ones, remember those real tangible losses.**

3.8: Creating a Lifestyle That Will Foster Your Goals

All of this comes down to helping you accomplish your goals. Stop creating tradeoffs with your time and know that if you make the effort, your lifestyle **will** set you up for success.

As with every change in your life, it is best to start out small. Be mindful of the traps and habits you are falling into and change them slowly. Don't go out tomorrow and try to walk 20,000 steps, meditate for 3 hours, and catch up on all the sleep you have lost. *It won't work.*

However, do write down things you want to improve in your lifestyle. Start with small steps. Write down three strategies or changes that you will implement into your lifestyle ***tomorrow***.

They could be as simple as taking a three-minute break every hour at work to clear your mind, but list them below and why they will help you accomplish your goals:

<u>Strategy or Change</u>   <u>Why It **Will** Contribute to Your Goals</u>

1. _____   _____

                              _____

                              _____

2. _____   _____

                              _____

                              _____

3. _____   _____

                              _____

                              _____

Create minute changes that will become habits. Eventually

you won't even realize that you have cut the time you sit per day in

half or that your morning and nightly rituals have become

engrained routines. Equate it to the big picture.

Realize that you need to change your lifestyle to accomplish your goals. If you don't, then you can't be surprised or blame anyone else when those goals pass you by. Create a sense of purpose with your lifestyle. **Know that you're improving yourself and that it will directly lead to success in the future.**

Finally, have fun with it. You should not dread sleeping more, better posture, stress relief, moving, your routines, or living a more natural, scenic life. These are part of being human! These should be embraced and enjoyed. Make them fun and dive into the vastness of your capabilities.

Key Takeaways:

- **Start with small changes in your lifestyle that will blossom and make a huge difference as they become daily habits.**

- **Enjoy being human and all of the wonderful lifestyle characteristics that go with it.**

Chapter 4: Nutrition - Keep It Simple Stupid

Nutrition is incredibly important. We digest over a thousand grams of food every single day. In fact, the food and liquids you digest are the *only things* you are **guaranteed** to put thousands of grams of inside your body every day.

Think about that for a second.

I am always so perplexed when people doubt that food is one of the single biggest influencers in their health. No one wants to point to bad food as the culprit for any disease or illness from cancer to a stroke. To put it in layman terms, those diseases occur in the tissue, cells, and organs that are internally contained within your body. What is the only thing that you put thousands of grams of into your body every day?

Food.

Ergo, what influences those tissues, cells, and organs the most?

Food!

We need to start giving food the importance it deserves. Food impacts your mental, emotional, and physical well-being on a daily basis. Treat food with respect and you will be respecting your body, mind, and goals.

You can't expect to eat processed crap and accomplish your goals. You will not be mentally sharp, physically energized or emotionally stable. Food is what keeps us running! Without food and water, we are *screwed*.

Think of the last time you felt run down and physically or emotionally drained, what was your diet like during this time? What kinds of food were you eating?

If you told me you were only eating whole foods, quality proteins, and several serving of vegetables and fruit per day, I would say bravo and we could confidently say your diet was not a factor. If that is not the case, then it is clear your diet was a contributing factor to the way you felt.

Whenever I ask someone why they don't eat as well as they should, they usually reply something like this, "I'm going to eat what I enjoy, and if I die early, well then I die early."

Two problems with this: first, they're **ass_um**ing good foods (remember not healthy) can't be just as tasty as processed garbage. Second, why would you not want to feel and perform your best?

The first problem is largely due to not experimenting with whole foods and the right ingredients in the kitchen, this is an easy fix. The second part I *never* understand.

Why would you not want to be able to do your *best* work?

Why would you not want to have *as much energy as possible* to experience everything you can in life?

Why would you not want to have the *best* life possible?

If you have absolutely no aspirations in life, you don't care about your wealth, health, happiness, or love and are just coasting by until your death, then the above answer is completely fine. If that is not what you want out of life, <u>then what the fuck are you talking about</u>!

If you want to achieve your goals, if you want a better life, if you want the best life possible for your children and family, then **wake the Hell up** and make the constant connection that food affects everything you do in life. *Not just physically*, but **mentally** and **emotionally** as well.

Nutrition doesn't have to be hard. In reality it is very simple. It has only become difficult in the last 50 years. Why is that? Barry Schwartz summarized this best in *The Paradox of Choice*.

We have *too many damn choices* in the grocery store.

Aisles filled with hundreds of different jars of sauces, snacks, and drinks. Even when it comes to good foods (see what I did there), like produce, you have a huge choice of vegetables and fruits that are always available even when they aren't in season. You have every piece of animal meat you could ever want and crops grown from all over the world.

Then you have diets constantly thrown in your face:

Paleo.

Gluten-free.

Low fat.

Carnivorous.

Ketogenic.

Vegetarian.

Diary-free.

Atkins, and it goes on and on.

Our caveman brains become *paralyzed*. No wonder everyone is confused, every diet tells you their diet is the only one that is correct and every other diet is **wrong**. With so many conflicting ideologies people can't choose and usually end up failing; eating whatever is easy and convenient.

We need to get rid of all the noise and get back to the basics. We will do this by simplifying your food choices and following a few simple principles that will cement long lasting habits, instead of the short-term, impossible to follow and extremely strict, guideline diets.

Diets will **never** work, understand this. I don't care if it is a celebrity diet, some trendy no-fat, no-carb diet, a cleanse, whatever it is, these are short-term band-aids that will leave you exactly where you started. The only way to be successful with nutrition is to instill *good eating habits* which will eventually become intuitive.

Key Takeaways:

- **Food is one of the single biggest influencers in your health.**

- **Cut through the paradox of choice and make food simple again with habits, not diets.**

- **Diets will never work! NEVER!**

4.1: The Secret of Nutrition

Do you want to know the secret of nutrition? Well here it is: we don't know that much about it. We don't. We know the basics and are doing studies every day to learn more, but we are far from mastering nutrition. Why isn't everyone a vegetarian? Why isn't everyone on the mountain dog diet?

Because every, single, person, is **different**.

We have different genetics.

 Different lives.

Different taste buds.

Different digestive enzymes.

Different goals.

All of us humans are vastly different. There will never be a blanket diet that will work for everyone. Anyone who touts a diet as a cure all or the perfect way to eat, is a scam artist. This is because anyone in the fitness and health industry with any knowledge knows what I stated above is true, so they are selling their product in spite of this, and *tricking you* into believing it is perfect for you.

A constant theme in the health world is getting the *"best"* product. We want the *"best"* fat burning workout. The *"best"* weight-loss diet. This is impossible. Unless you have machines and researchers monitoring your vitals and blood work at all hours of the day, *you will never figure this out*.

In reality, as long as we are incorporating good nutritional principles and activity habits, we will lose weight and be healthy. Once you get rid of trying to have the "best" program, then you can actually start focusing on doing things you like and creating good habits which in turn will get you the results you want much faster than constantly stressing out about having the *optimal* program.

I am not throwing a diet at you.

I am giving you guidelines of large scale principles that are proven to work. Most of what I'm going to tell you is pretty basic, I just put it together in an easy to understand and easy to implement fashion.

When it comes to your food journey I can't tell you exactly what you should eat, no one can, **except for you**. I don't know what tastes, textures, and combinations you like. <u>Only you do</u>.

I am going to give you a broad foundation, it is then your turn to chisel away and create your masterpiece. I will make this easier for you. The strategies I lay out really do work, but at the same time you have to be accountable, explorative, and take charge of your journey through food. The cats out of the bag, now let's cook it: figuratively of course.

Key Takeaways:

- **Every single human being is different, there will never be a "best" or blanket diet that works.**

- **We will create healthy nutritional habits; however, you must tailor your nutrition to fit your life and preferences.**

- **The only person who knows exactly what you should eat, is YOU!**

4.2: Cook Damnit!

If you're a grown adult reading this and you don't know how to cook for yourself, that is a *damn shame and needs to change*. Food is **primal**.

Hunting, gathering, and cooking are survival instincts and we get pleasure from doing them. They satisfy our needs while also flourishing us with accomplishment.

You need to have pride in what you eat and how you obtain it. Having food set down in front of you does nothing. In this scenario, you're worth less: you're an able-bodied, intellectually minded human being yet you're unable to make your own food and you're taking away a pivotal part of being human. You don't even need to go out to hunt or gather your food anymore. Food is now packaged and ready for you, all you need to do is cook and create.

Cooking is essential to health.

You are **not in control** of *your goals* or *your destiny*, when you go out to eat at a restaurant. Someone is deciding what options you have and how those options are made, you're simply a

puppet.

Food at your typical restaurant is drenched in unhealthy oils and butters which skyrocket the calories. It has preservatives, other unnatural characteristics, and portion sizes that are usually completely out of whack. You need to make the change right now to make eating out a luxury. It should not occur often, once a week or less.

There is no argument to cooking your own food. It is cheaper than even the lowest quality fast food, it is healthier, it will create a skill that will develop you as a person, it makes you accountable for what you're eating, and it is fun!

Cooking is incredibly simple. To cook our fresh, gourmet meals we will simply follow the good food outline below on what carbs, fats, and proteins to buy from the grocery store. From here, we will need a pot, a couple of non-stick pans, and the seasonings and herbs of your choosing.

I was always confused when other college students would come into my dorm and say something like, "Wow, that's amazing. How do you know how to cook?"

Well you see I put a pan on the stove. Put the stove on medium. Put some olive oil in the pan. Put in the food. Put some herbs and spices on the food. Now I watch the food until it is done! It really is not that difficult, but I would hear time and time again,

"I could never do that, I'm a terrible cook!" Don't create self-doubt, **I promise you can do this**.

It is time to get excited about cooking and cooking good food! We live in the most amazing generation of information where everything you could ever want is right at your fingertips. You can YouTube any cooking technique you please.

Want to watch Gordon Ramsey effortlessly cut up a whole chicken? Boom, YouTube.

Don't know how to create a wine reduction sauce? Boom, YouTube.

Don't know how to cut up a mango? I think you get the point.

You have all of the best culinary minds at the tips of your fingers, utilize them! You can find delicious recipes made with only good ingredients anywhere online. Search for recipes online with the ingredients you have.

If you have a more concrete idea of what you want, you can search for specific recipes like, "Best bolognaise recipe ever," or "Making authentic, stir fry teriyaki chicken like a boss."

Have fun with cooking, get friends involved, roommates, your family and your kids! Play some music, dance and sing while you cook, think about how delicious this meal is going to be.

Create suspense!

Think of how proud you're of yourself for being able to learn this skill and create a masterpiece you will perfect. Did we already talk about attitude being everything? Good, I digress.

Key Takeaways:

- With cooking you can control the quality of your ingredients and exactly what goes into your food.

- Treat cooking as an adventure and your time in the kitchen might possibly be the most fun you have all day!

4.3: The 80/20 Rule

An easy and effective way to start taking control of your nutritional habits is with the 80/20 rule. Most people go crazy when starting a diet, because they go from eating McDonalds and Twinkies one day, to eating nothing but raw kale covered in sesame seeds the next.

No shit this isn't going to work long-term!

Over time, we do want to get rid of the McDonalds and Twinkies, but it isn't happening **day one**. The 80/20 rule is a great way to create a ***balance*** of eating mostly good foods, while still indulging in some of the bad foods that you are accustomed to.

It will look like this: for every 80 things I eat that will help me accomplish my goal, I can eat 20 things that will not help my goal.

Or more simply put an 8:2 ratio. This principal can also be used in things like your career, getting better at a hobby, savings, etc.

For the diet portion, you will keep track of your decisions like a game. Every serving of a food you eat has to go in one column or the other and you have to track it. Here is an example of using the 80/20 rule at a meal: Breakfast - Cooking eggs in olive oil, with sautéed spinach, a kiwi, and a SMALL bowl of Lucky Charms.

Start with two columns:

This **Will** Help My Goals	This Will **NOT** Help My Goals
1. Olive Oil	1. Small Bowl of Lucky Charms
2. Eggs	
3. Spinach	
4. Kiwi	

The olive oil, eggs, spinach, and kiwi, count as 4 points since these are great food items that will help you accomplish your goals, keep you nutritiously satisfied for hours to come, and provide you with the energy to tackle anything your morning brings.

That's amazing!

Now that small bowl of Lucky Charms is loaded with unhealthy chemicals, preservatives, bad flour, sugar, oils, etc. So this is not going to help you accomplish your goals. This will go in the opposite column.

However, you stayed on track! With this example you are at a 4 to 1 ratio right now which is where you need to be to stay at an 8 to 2 ratio. You mostly ate a nutritionally dense breakfast and at the same time you had that little comfort food you are used to, so you didn't turn your world upside down. You will put every food you eat in one column or the other.

It is pretty simple, any food made by man that is heavily processed, will go in the second column, which is **not** helping you accomplish your goals.

Very lightly processed foods like 100% whole wheat pasta or anything that naturally comes from the Earth, is a whole food and unprocessed, will be in column one which will be _helping_ you accomplish your goals.

Whole foods are fruits, vegetables, nuts, seeds, meats, eggs, or oils which naturally exists on the Earth. We will go into more detail on good foods below to give you a better idea of what you should be eating.

With this rule we need to keep it in proportion of serving sizes. One carrot is **NOT** equivalent to a Big Mac. There is no perfect way to scale this, so you have to be mindful and realistic with yourself.

This is why I noted a small bowl of Lucky Charms in the example above. If this was a regular sized bowl, it may be two points in the column of foods not helping your goals. If it were a large bowl, three, and so on.

If you eat an entire fast food or crappy meal, then you will have to put it in proportion to the food you ate through your entire day. That means if you had three meals that day, the fast food meal would be equivalent to 1/3 of your day's points and this is only the case if all three meals were roughly the same size. A ratio of 1:3 is not staying on target.

When applying this strategy, it is much easier to have the 20% of the *shitty foods* be dispersed throughout your day. Having just a small piece of comfort food a couple times per day will satisfy your cravings better and be healthier than cramming all of your bad foods into a cheat meal for the day or **even worse**, a cheat day for the week.

Cheat meals and cheat days are an incredibly unhealthy habit both physically and psychologically. Having cheat meals and cheat days creates an unnatural restriction on the majority of your day or week, while encouraging a mentally-scaring binge at certain intervals.

These binges crash your metabolism, insulin levels, and spirit. This is an incredibly unhealthy habit that should *never* be used, especially when trying to lose weight.

The point system comes back to taking responsibility. You want to decrease the 80/20 rule as time goes on and better eating habits are developed. After 6 months or so you want to make it a 90/10 rule. After a year, a 95/5 rule. With time nutrition does become intuitive and you will not even notice you are eating this way. You will enjoy eating good foods and your good habits will become cemented into your life.

The 80/20 rule always comes down to owning your decisions and actions, as well as tracking your columns. No extreme restrictiveness for six days followed by a day of binge eating crap. No counting calories or macros, just simply a mark per each food in one column or the other.

Key Takeaways:

- **Utilize the 80/20 rule to create balance in your nutrition with healthy staples and the occasional comfort food you are used to.**

- **AVOID cheat meals and cheat days like the plague, these are unhealthy habits that will damage you physically and psychologically.**

4.4: Know Thy Serving Size

It should be of no surprise to anyone that American portions and sizes are skewed compared to the rest of the world. We **LOVE** our non-produce carbs and meats, oh boy, do we.

Look at the typical menu: <u>16 ounce steaks</u> or <u>half a chicken</u> as your protein portion. Look at the typical plate, it is usually entirely covered in a base of heavy carbohydrates. There is usually an entire layer of rice covering every inch of the plate or pasta that is piled high and enough for a family of four. What are you not going to see?

A heaping piles of vegetables.

Usually the three baby carrots and two broccoli florets drenched in butter will not even equal a *half serving* of vegetables. This is something that is entrenched in our society: bigger is better.

Everywhere from televisions to fireworks displays, we are always trying to make things as big as possible. The majority of the restaurant industry has taken advantage of this novelty.

The average person is more concerned with the amount they are eating rather than the quality of food they are eating. For a sedentary person, it takes much less food than you would think to satisfy their bodies' needs.

There are a large multitude of studies involving all sorts of animal species from dogs to monkeys to fruit flies, proving that eating less prolongs life.[37,38] By lowering the caloric intake of the animals' diets by 30-40% the animals all live 20-40% longer. Many scientists hypothesize this is to be true in humans and have called this the ultimate anti-aging serum.

We should not be eating past fullness and should only be eating when we are actually hungry. Whenever your hunger is satisfied, stop eating!

Unless you're an world-class athlete or lean person trying to build muscle, eating past fullness is not good for you. You should restrain yourself when you are full even if your plate is not cleared. There can always be leftovers.

This is a healthy habit that will go a long way. As you start to focus more and more on eating whole foods you will actually need fewer calories overtime to fill you up, which will create that natural anti-aging effect.

The typical American diet consists of way too many simple carbs like pasta, rice, and bread, too many low-quality meats, too many processed snacks foods full of sugar and crappy ingredients, and not nearly enough fruits and vegetables. So what's the plan?

Cut out everything but broccoli!

I'M KIDDING! *Don't do that.*

We simply want to create a **balanced** diet. This doesn't mean cutting out pasta or chicken it just means eating good quality food, while making the amount of pasta we eat, equal to the amount of chicken we eat, equal to the amount of produce we eat. Balanced. The easiest way to create balance is through serving sizes. There is an incredibly easy way to start eating healthy portions and it is...

Wait for the shock.... By cooking!

When you're cooking all you have to do is look on the side of the pasta box, olive oil jar, or spinach bag and it will tell you how much a serving is. You hold all the power mighty one! If you have a lone piece of fruit or produce without such writing a 20 second Google search will answer your serving size question.

A decent rule of thumb is that a serving of meat or fish is four ounces, which is a quarter of a pound or a small handful. A package of meat or fish will always tell you the weight. If you have a 12-ounce piece of mahi mahi, then cut it into thirds and each third is one serving size.

A serving of fruits or vegetables is usually about a large handful, which is much bigger than most people think.

A serving of pasta, rice, or beans, what is usually the largest part of the plate, is only about a ¼ cup dry. This is much smaller than most people think.

When we implement healthy serving sizes it should not be stressful! We are not going to be counting calories. We just want balanced meals. If you are making a stir fry dish this would mean per every 4 ounces or small handful of beef, chicken, or shrimp you use, you would use a ¼ cup of rice, and a decent sized handful of vegetables.

That is <u>balance</u>.

Zen if you would.

You don't need to worry about balancing good fats since you will get plenty of these with your healthy cooking oils, the cuts of meat you will be choosing, the fresh fish you will incorporate into your meals, and from your good foods in-between meals like avocados and nuts.

This is relatively easy: your food will fit on a regular sized dining plate for any meal and it will be divided equally between proteins, produce (vegetables and fruits), and the non-produce carbohydrates like pasta, rice, beans, or bread.

This is the simplest way to have a nutritional balance with an American diet. Over time this is will become intuitive. You won't even have to think about it, these habits will become ingrained behaviors.

Key Takeaways:

- **Learn to cook with proportional serving sizes to balance your plate and your nutrition.**

- **Create the habit to stop eating once you are full, there can always be leftovers!**

4.5: Less is More

When it comes to less is more I'm talking about processed food. Whether it is nuts, bread, or any food item you eat, a good rule of thumb is the *less* processed the food, *the better*. The least amount of ingredients, the better the food will be. The closer the food is to its' natural state, the better.

For example, it only takes four ingredients to make bread and the only bread you should buy is bread made with simple ingredients like water, yeast, flour, and salt. Do not buy anything with high fructose corn syrup, hydrogenated oils that aren't necessary, or ingredients that you have no idea what they are.

It is helpful to go back through our history and remember what the human species' natural diet is. If you take out the last 50 to 100 years, for hundreds of thousands of years we always ate the same things: meat, fish, eggs, produce, seeds, nuts, and naturally farmed crops like rice, wheat, and corn.

There were no heavily processed foods, no additives, preservatives, pesticides, herbicides, artificial ingredients, etc. So for 99.99% of our entire existence we never ingested these things.

Yes, the human body is amazing. It can be severely abused for decades and still survive.

It can deal with a large amount of antibiotics. It can also handle a decent amount of chemicals like pesticides and preservatives.

Does that mean these practices are healthy? **No**.

Does that mean eating those artificial ingredients and chemicals is going to help you accomplish your goals? **Absolutely not**.

It is helpful to understand all of the engineered, processed foods in our stores today are not natural or meant to be part of our biology. You will limit processed foods from your diet by sticking to your healthy eating habits. By being mindful of the ingredients in your food and the quality of that food, we will limit the ingestion of these shitty ingredients.

When making your food choices at the grocery store you want to stick closer to whole foods that are natural, like grass-fed beef and dairy products, animals that aren't treated with antibiotics or hormones, and produce that is organic or not as affected by pesticides and herbicides. Don't worry, we will also make this affordable. First, we have a few more principles to cover.

Key Takeaway:

- **You want to simplify the amount of ingredients in your food and use ingredients that are more naturally procured.**

4.6: Whole Foods, not Half

Look at many of the healthier diets out there: paleo, vegetarian, vegan, carnivorous, mountain dog, etc. What do they all revolved around?

<u>Eating whole foods</u>!

I have seen countless vegan and vegetarian blood results that look excellent. I have worked with athletes on all animal-product diets (only eating eggs, meat, animal fats, and fish), and they also have blood results that are amazing. Everyone is different and the human digestive system is flexible. This is why we want to customize.

Don't become a _cult diet_ member!

However, with all of these diets that we see great health results from they all have the common link of revolving around whole foods. Foods that naturally occur in this world whether they are vegetables, fruits, nuts, seeds, oils, fish, eggs, or meats.

Jack Lalanne, one of the pioneers of health and fitness was

famous for saying, "If man made it, don't eat it." The problems with food arise when it is heavily processed. Grass-fed beef has an amazing nutrient profile, but heavily processed, chemically loaded pepperoni does not.

Is that really surprising? *It shouldn't be.*

The more you stick to a diet of whole foods, no matter what kinds, the better off you will be. In the 80/20 rule, whole foods fall under the first category and are foods that will **help** us accomplish our goals. By eating whole foods more often you will actually need less food to keep yourself full, plus you will satisfy your body and mind more nutritiously which will make your goals even more attainable.

Key Takeaway:

- **Focus on eating mostly whole foods and you will be just fine, remember health habits not diets.**

4.7: On the Go and the Luxuries of Life

If you are not cooking and creating your own food, then you can't control what is in it. This is always something to keep in mind whether you travel frequently or you go out to eat with friends for dinner on certain occasions.

Even though you may not be in control you can still make the most of the options you have. This includes eating as many whole foods as possible that are processed as little as possible and picking options that will help balance your plate.

Oils, butters, sauces, and cooking techniques are mainly what creates unhealthy food in restaurants. Nonetheless, it is impossible to control _their_ cooking techniques or the kind of oil _they_ use to cook food.

You can only make the best decisions with the options in front of you. Ultimately, you need to treat eating out for what it was originally meant to be: _a luxury_. Sticking to whole foods, balancing your plate and serving sizes, while using the 80/20 rule will help you make better decisions, but even those healthy eating habits will not produce the same results as you cooking your own food at home.

At the same token, this is not a time to stress!

You are creating nutritional principles instead of a diet for a reason, so that those good decisions become natural. Be aware of what you're eating and try to cut back on eating out when possible. When you're out, you can indulge in pieces, but be mindful not to go overboard.

If there is an incredible German chocolate cake on the menu and this is your favorite dessert, then get it! Just be mindful of the 80/20 rule and focus on eating mostly whole foods throughout the other portions of this day.

Key Takeaway:

- **Eating out should be treated as a luxury, but when you do eat out you should not stress, simply stick to the healthy nutritional habits above and be mindful when you do indulge.**

4.8: Meal Time Foods vs. Snack Foods

We have this idea in America that we have snack foods and we have meal-time foods.

They can't be both! We eat meals to *fill us up*. We eat snacks to *hold* ourselves over.

Most times we eat snacks attempting to sequester our hunger until dinner, but these snacks are usually not very nutrient dense and are heavily processed, so our bodies naturally crave more and become hungry again.

So you eat another snack.

Still hungry?

Have another!

It really is a vicious cycle. Before you know it, you have eaten hundreds of calories of crappy foods that did **nothing** for you. This is what makes the snack industry so successful. Would they make money if five potato chips actually filled you up? **No**.

Why not eat snacks that actually fill you up? How would you

do that? You will accomplish this by eating the same whole foods for your meals and snacks.

We treat food and time with this weird mutual exclusiveness. Americans often think eggs and fruit can only be eaten during breakfast. In reality, eggs aren't just a breakfast food, neither is fruit. You can eat anything at any time of the day! In Japanese culture, it is common to have soup, vegetables, and sashimi or sushi for breakfast. You can do this too if you wanted!

You can eat half a chicken thigh with some guacamole and salsa on top as a snack at 10:30 am, it doesn't have to be at a dinner or lunch meal. If you were to eat this instead of all of your crappy snack foods, then you would actually be full afterwards!

With this delicious snack you would be getting in a couple dozen grams of protein, good fats, several produce items, and the same amount of calories as a shitty snack pack that comes dry, tasteless, and in a box!

You might actually have energy after eating this instead of

crashing and looking at the clock every 5 minutes, begging for lunch to come.

When it comes to eating healthy snacks all it takes is cooking a little extra good food a day or two beforehand. That way, when you're on the go you have food already cooked and you can throw together a tasty combination in a short amount of time. This only takes a little extra planning and preparation.

Stop categorizing food as meal time foods or snack foods. They are all the same: **food**. Let's explore some good foods that you should be eating.

Key Takeaways:

- **You cannot categorize food; it is all simply food.**

- **Eat the same foods you would during meal times also at your snack times to satisfy your hunger and your body's nutritional needs.**

4.9: The Good Fats

I said we are going to make this simple right? Do you trust me? Of course you do!

Ok, your good fats are going to include the oils you cook with, which will be olive oil, unrefined extra virgin coconut oil, or grass-fed butter. Your fats will also include nuts, animal fats, and avocados. Animal fats will be included in the cuts of meat we choose or the fish we eat in the protein section. Avocados are produce so this is a win-win item.

As for the nuts, you want to keep these as least processed as possible. Roasted and salted are ok, but you don't want candied or flavored nuts. Raw nuts aren't for everyone, most people need a little salt for taste, but I would recommend them.

The oils you cook with are going to be the most important part of this section. Where most restaurants and people go wrong is by using crappy, high calorie, low nutrient oils in their cooking.

You are going to cook exclusively with olive oil, unrefined extra virgin coconut oil, and grass-fed butter. There is a *ridiculous* amount of scientific studies on olive oil that prove its' amazing heart healthy benefits.[31] This should be a staple in your cooking.

You should use extra virgin olive oil, as it less refined and closer to its natural state. When buying olive oil, organic is the best kind, but it is much more expensive. The next best alternative is to get cold pressed olive oil which is lightly processed naturally. If this is out of your budget, focus on getting pure olive oil. Sometimes companies will try to blend other oils in there with olive oil. Be aware of that and go for 100% olive oil.

When cooking with olive oil <u>always </u>keep the heat at medium or below this way the oil will remain stable and below its' smoke point. This is a helpful tip, because unless you are trying to sear meat there really isn't much else you should be cooking above medium. Medium does the job just fine and is much easier to handle for less experienced cooks. Side note, if you are trying to sear meat use one of the other two oils below.

Unrefined extra virgin coconut oil is another fantastic oil with many great heart healthy benefits. It has a slightly sweeter taste and compliments many dishes wonderfully. Usually this oil is sold in organic form, and the price between non-organic and organic is pretty similar.

We want to make sure this oil is unrefined and extra virgin as this means it is minimally processed and in a better state. Now that coconut oil has finally become mainstream, rejoice, as it should be easy to find at any supermarket.

Lastly, we have grass-fed butter. Butter normally gets a bad rap, but this is because most butter is heavily processed and not from healthy cows. You'll see a trend with our cow products, we want them all grass-fed. Why?

We go back to *natural biology*.

A Cow's natural diet is grass, not grain and corn. Just with any animal, their diet affects everything from their organ health, to the nutrients in their milk, and even the omega-3 content in their muscle. Grass-fed cows produce much ***more nutrient dense*** and healthier forms of milk and meat.

Grass-fed cows contain a great ratio of omega-3 to omega-6 fatty acids. I could explain the difference and go into detail of long chain vs. short chain, yadi, yadi, yada.

All you really need to know is that omega-3's are our best source of fats when it comes to heart health. Omega-6's are also great for many functions, but with all things in life, balance is important. Omega-6's will actually destroy omega-3's at the cellular level if you eat too many foods with Omega-6's.[32,33]

Omega-3's are much harder to get in the Western diet as they primarily exist in grass-fed animal products, certain seeds, fish like salmon, tuna, sardines, or eggs. Omega-6s occur in most other foods besides produce and are heavily present in badly processed oils, wheat products, snack foods, etc.

Shit, more detail than I should have gone into.

To sum it up, by eating grass-fed products you are keeping a healthy, balanced omega ratio, while also eating more nutrient dense food. Bam, easy answer.

By cooking with healthy oils, having grass-fed products and fish be staples in your diet, and eating healthy snacks like nuts and avocados, you will be getting plenty of healthy fats in your diet which will improve your body composition, heart, and overall health.

Key Takeaways:

- **Utilize olive oil, coconut oil, and grass-fed butter as your healthy cooking oils.**

- **Integrate minimally processed nuts, avocados, fish, and a variety of cuts of meat to get a wide variety of tasty healthy fats in your nutrition.**

4.10: Carbohydrates – Our First Love

I think one of my favorite lines in any movie was in *Austin Powers: Goldmember* when Fat Bastard said, "Carbs are the enemy." The context was perfect.

This is how many Americans think, but this is only the case because our culture has abused carbs so badly and we constantly gorge on them. Almost all processed foods are mainly carbs: chips, crackers, bread, wheat products, granola bars, you name it. Most American's live a *heavily* carb dominated diet.

Carbs are not your enemy; <u>the way you eat them is</u>! Most people don't think of fresh vegetables and fruits as carbohydrates, but that's what most of them purely are. Fruits and vegetables contain fewer grams of carbs and calories, but many more nutrients and vitamins. You need these in your diet! Eat as many as possible.

The new trend is that fruit is bad! Fruit has sugar and that sugar will kill you! First of all, sugar in fruit is much different than sugar in candy, both in quality and quantity. The body digests sugar in fruit much more slowly as it is a long-chain carbohydrate and contains many other vitamins, minerals, and components to digest. Secondly, fruits and vegetables are much more than just fiber and food sources, they are *disease fighters* and *preventers*.

Kiwi has large amounts of glutathione which <u>prevents</u> gene mutation and cancer.

Blueberries have more antioxidants than any other produce item, which <u>get rid of</u> free radicals and waste in cells.

Carrots and sweet potatoes have huuuuggge amounts of beta carotene which is proven to <u>prevent</u> cardiovascular disease.[40,41]

Broccoli and many other veggies contain isothiocyanates, which has been proven through research to <u>kill</u> cancer cells.[35]

Food is your *medicine*.

There are so many benefits to eating produce, take advantage of all of them by eating as much produce as possible. These incredible foods will boost your body and mind to help you conquer all of your goals.

When eating produce, it is best to buy organic. If this is not in your budget then I suggest buying seasonal produce as it is cheaper, and sticking to the list of the clean fifteen and the dirty dozen. This is a listed produced by the Environmental Working Group and is updated each year.[45]

The dirty dozen details which produce items are most affected by pesticides, herbicides, and other chemical means used in conventional farming. The produce in the dirty dozen you should try to buy organic whenever possible

The clean fifteen, are the produce items least affected by those same chemicals. You can buy these produce items conventionally grown without worrying as much.

Combine these lists with eating items that are in season and locally grown, and your budget will be much more robust. Below are the full lists of the clean fifteen and dirty dozen courtesy of the Environmental Working Group (EWG):[45]

The Clean Fifteen	The Dirty Dozen
1. Avocados	1. Strawberries
2. Sweet Corn	2. Apples
3. Pineapples	3. Nectarines
4. Cabbage	4. Peaches
5. Sweet Peas Frozen	5. Celery
6. Onions	6. Grapes
7. Asparagus	7. Cherries
8. Mangos	8. Spinach
9. Papayas	9. Tomatoes
10. Kiwi	10. Sweet Bell Peppers
11. Eggplant	11. Cherry Tomatoes
12. Honeydew Melon	12. Cucumbers
13. Grapefruit	Bonus Items Dirty Dozen:

14. Cantaloupe   + Hot Peppers

15. Cauliflower   + Kale/Collard Greens

When picking produce and crops at the grocery store you should also stick to Non-GMO or Non-Genetically Modified Organisms, whenever possible. This is especially necessary when it comes to corn, soy, and wheat products which are usually the staple crops for genetic modification.

The science behind genetically modified crops is still heavily debated; however, what we do know is these crops are ***extremely damaging*** to the environment and are typically less nutrient dense.[46] These practices are destroying bee populations which are vitally important for pollination and the entire ecosystem. Until the practices used in farming GMO crops are cleaned up, it is best to steer clear of these products.

Lastly, frozen fruits and vegetables will stretch your budget to the max. You can buy all sorts of frozen produce, especially when the produce item you are looking for is out of season and will not be fresh. The only characteristics to be wary of when buying frozen produce are hidden ingredients. The only ingredient on the package should be the produce item!

All too often in frozen food items companies will sneak harmful hidden ingredients into the food, be cognizant of this and always check the ingredient labels.

In order to balance your plate correctly, you will categorize carbs as those that are produce and those that are not.

Non-produce carbs are still healthy and great energy sources, but you want to balance them with your carbs that are produce to get the full benefits of a balanced diet.

With carbs like pasta, rice, lentils and beans (also a good protein source), go organic if possible. For these carbs, the difference in price between conventional and organic products is usually <u>very small</u>. Always stick to products with the *least* amount of ingredients. There shouldn't be anything else on the ingredient list besides the actual crop. Buy these crops raw and dry to make sure they are in their natural state and minimally processed.

If you're a bread lover stick to bread with very simple ingredients: water, yeast, salt, flour is typically all you really need. This would be an excellent time to learn how to make your own bread whether it be whole wheat or sourdough.

This is incredibly fun especially when you get loved ones involved, it is cheaper, and you can add whatever spices and additions you'd like to satisfy any of your taste buds' cravings. Plus, how good is fresh bread straight out of the oven, to die for!

Remember, when it comes to carbs you want to stick mostly to the whole foods listed above. Heavily processed carbs are not going to do you any favors, and should be kept to the 20% section of the 80/20 rule.

Even food items that seem healthy like organic granola bars are usually full of sugar and processed simple carbs which will be burned by your body extremely fast leaving behind little nutritional value. Instead focus on filling your snacks with more complex and nutritional whole food carbohydrates like produce, rice, beans, and lentils. These will keep you full throughout the day and busy as a bee, ready for whatever life throws at you!

Key Takeaways:

- **Balance your produce and non-produce carbohydrates to create a well-rounded nutrition.**

- **When it comes to produce buy organic when possible, stick to the list of the clean fifteen and the dirty dozen, and buy local produce to expand your budget.**

- **When it comes to non-produce carbohydrates stick to raw and dry, organic, and minimally or unprocessed foods.**

4.11: Protein for the Soul

Protein is a pretty simple topic. Your main proteins will come down to eggs, fish, dairy and meat. There is protein in beans, lentils, seeds, and other foods, however, if you are like most Americans you're not a vegetarian. There is also no concrete evidence that a vegetarian based diet is better than one with healthy protein choices from good sources like we will discuss below.

It is great to eat a wide variety of whole foods, in saying this, lentils, beans, seeds, and vegetarian protein sources are great foods. If you enjoy those foods implement them into your diet. I would encourage everyone to try having a few vegetarian meals per week as many of these are delicious and will enhance your culinary experience while letting you try even more whole foods. However, for most Americans eggs, fish, dairy products, and meats will be your *staple* proteins.

Let's start with eggs.

Eggs are a very complete food with tons of vitamins and minerals. They have good omega-3 fatty acids, as well as complete proteins with bioavailable B Vitamins. This means the form of B vitamins in eggs, as well as those found in meat and fish, are very easy for the body to absorb. Eggs also contain cholesterol which is *incredibly* important for everything from organ health to hormonal health.

It was just announced by the American Heart Association that in many cases the cholesterol in food does not adversely affect the cholesterol in blood. There are also studies showing tribal cultures that eat enormous amounts of cholesterol, *more than 10x* the cholesterol of the average American, and these indigenous people have amazingly healthy cholesterol levels in their blood which are rarely seen in the Western world.[34]

There are a multitude of studies showing tribal cultures who eat vast amounts of saturated fats and they have no presence of stroke or heart disease either.[42]

Rest easy, cholesterol **won't** kill you neither will saturated fats. On the contrary, *they are quite good for you and necessary nutrients when consumed from good sources.*

Now back to eggs.

The more orange an egg yolk is, the more chlorophyll is in the yolk, which means the hens were fed a better diet. This will make the eggs more nutrient dense. With that said, your first option would be to get organic, pasture raised eggs, but these are also the most expensive.

The next best option would be to get eggs from vegetarian fed hens and with the **certified humane seal of approval** on the package label. This label means the hens are raised in better conditions. These are still more expensive probably around $3.50-4 a dozen.

The final option would be to get eggs that are from vegetarian fed hens without any antibiotics or hormones. These are usually around $2-2.50 a dozen.

Be aware: the cage free label does not mean much anymore since the federal guidelines for being cage free are so loose. Many cage free egg companies still overcrowd their hens in small pens without sunlight. *Don't get fooled by this label*!

Mooo!

Dairy is a complicated subject. Many people are lactose intolerant even to a small degree, so <u>you are the only person</u> who can know if dairy is for you. If you can tolerate dairy and enjoy it, then stick to dairy products from grass-fed cows not treated with any antibiotics or hormones. When it comes to yogurt and other dairy products like kefir, minimize the ingredients and watch for high levels of added sugar. If grass-fed dairy products are not an option stick to dairy that is from cows ***not*** treated with any antibiotics or hormones.

We'll move to the ocean for our next protein source: fish. Fish contains an amazing amount of omega-3 fatty acids and large amounts of protein topping **20-25 grams per serving**. This is almost as much protein as a serving of steak!

You want to buy **wild** fish. Wild fish live in their natural environments with their natural diets. Farm raised fish are fed pellets of usually *grain and corn that are dyed with coloring*. Farm raised fish are substantially **less** nutrient dense.

Wild fish like tuna, salmon, mahi mahi, snapper, mackerel, and sardines are great choices. You also can't go wrong with getting any wild fish that is caught <u>in season</u>.

Buying frozen wild seafood will help your budget stretch further. Wild scallops, shrimp, and other crustaceans are also great choices, but are usually a little more expensive depending on your location. Focus on the *seasonality* of your local seafood to get the best bang for your buck.

Meat, the king of the proteins in America. For beef and lamb, we want organic and grass-fed if possible, but as long as they are grass-fed we are happy. Grain fed cattle are inferior in the nutrients and ratios that we are looking for, plus these farming methods go against their natural biology.

It is hard to find organic or pasteur-raised chicken and pork, but this is the best quality of meat. We will settle for animals that are vegetarian fed as this will produce a better quality meat. For all meat we want to make sure it is antibiotic and hormone free.

This is no longer a dietary issue, but a real health hazard as **antibiotic resistant superbugs** are developing in animals due to the excess use of antibiotics. World governments are now getting involved to help stop the use of these malpractices.

This goes back to our natural talk, animals were raised without these malpractices for hundreds of thousands of years, they aren't necessary. Improvements in science and medicine are great, but we have used some of these improvements as blanket solutions for every issue even when they aren't necessary, which is why we are now having problems with these superbugs. Be a conscious consumer and avoid animals raised with these malpractices.

I digress.

Wild game is a terrific choice for meat as these animals live in their natural habitat and are **nutrient rich**. Many people aren't used to the gamey taste, but this can become a wonderful flavor with good cooking methods and seasonings.

No matter what kind of meat or fish you like, always try to switch it up and eat a wide variety. Let's talk about cuts of meat really quick. In America, for some reason we like the *least* flavor-full cuts of meat: chicken breast and filet mignon. Both cuts have almost no fat which is where a lot of flavor comes from and they are usually bland and dry.

It's pretty hard to cook a chicken breast just right. Your margin of error is so small from, "Ooh, I don't know that looks a little under done," to, "Well, now it's leather."

Explore different cuts of meat in different dishes to really develop your culinary side. Cuts like thighs, legs, and ribeyes are less popular alternatives with more flavor and moistness.

Explore!

Key Takeaways:

- **Stick to the quality suggestions above when purchasing eggs, fish, diary, and meat.**

- **Focus on animals that are raised the right way biologically and physically, for more nutrient dense food.**

4.12: Getting a Little Spicy and Saucy

Sauces are an obvious area where many people get into trouble. A salad isn't that great if it's *drenched* in ranch dressing. Herbs and spices in general, are much better than sauces.

It's hard to beat fresh basil on a pizza, hand-picked parsley on a spaghetti dish, or mouthwatering mint to compliment citrus notes in any meal. Not to mention the *natural low calorie aspect* of herbs and spices. Although, I know we love our sauces too, so let's discuss ways to pick good ones.

When picking sauces, go by ingredients, not phrases on the label.

Low-fat is usually code for, "We put a lot of other nasty shit in here to make this possible." A classic rule of thumb is to know the ingredients. If you don't know what many of them are, don't get the sauce. However, if you see a dressing with an ingredient label like this:

Olive oil, balsamic vinegar, mustard seed, sea salt, water, turmeric, honey, black pepper, and spices.

It is safe to assume you know all of these ingredients and this is a trustworthy dressing or sauce. I know *some* will argue just because you do not know what an ingredient is, that doesn't mean it is bad.

This is true, not *every* time is it bad, but in ***most cases***, it is.

Unless you want to put in the countless hours necessary to learn what every single artificial ingredient really is and what it does, then only getting foods with ingredients you know is a pretty good blanket rule for the average consumer.

The same rule applies to ingredients in seasoning mixes. If you see corn syrup, monosodium glutamate (MSG), or any other ingredient on the label do not buy it! There should only be spices and herbs on the label.

A healthy alternative for flavoring meals is salsa. This is a fantastic substitute that can be used in tons of dishes. It can even be blended to create a sauce-like consistency. Salsa is inexpensive even if it is an organic brand and it is a great sauce containing tons of spices, herbs, and actual produce.

As you go through this culinary experience try using less sauce over time. You need *much less* than you think you do when you use herbs and spices appropriately. Sauce is fine in moderation, but try to get better at using it for small tastes rather than *soaking* your food in it.

Key Takeaways:

- **Only pick sauces with ingredients you know.**

- **Take advantage of delicious herbs, spices, and salsas to create wonderful meals.**

- **Use sauce to compliment a meal, not overpower it.**

4.13: The Fountain of Youth

Ah, our thirst-quenchers. This is a touchy subject. With the dietary suggestions above I tried not to be restrictive. I wanted to give an outline of all of the foods you should try to eat the most of and knowledge of what food protocols are the best, even if you can't afford them right now.

Drinks are a different story mostly because of one kind: **soda**.

Sodas are pretty firmly rooted in American culture. Coke and Pepsi are almost as American as apple pie, maybe even more so today. Which is too bad, because they really are terrible for us.

Sodas and soda fountains back in the day, *were meant to be treats*. They were only meant to be had on special occasions, not every day occurrences. They also used better ingredients in the soda back then.

The average American drinks about 45 gallons of soda every year, that is over 18,000 grams of sugar. [14]

Holy shit is right.

Not to mention that soda literally does **nothing** good for you. The sugar spikes your insulin and equates to fat, this later results in crashes. Trust me, I really hate being restrictive.

I try to balance absolutely everything from lifestyle to activity to nutrition. Although, this is one thing we really should eliminate completely or treat it like it was meant to be, a **seldom** luxury.

Everything else, I am completely okay with in moderation. Hops in beer actually have quite a few health benefits, not to mention that alcohol is a natural blood thinner. Wine has antioxidants. Tea has many fantastic properties as does real coffee. Even 100% juices have important vitamins and minerals.

However, soda does not provide you any benefits. For God sakes, soda can clean a toilet because the acid will literally eat away at anything. What do you think it does to your insides, teeth, or health in general?

Unfortunately, I can't just limit this to soda anymore either as energy drinks, sports drinks, fruit juices that are not 100% juice, and even coffee-like drinks that are no longer recognizable as coffee are all filled with nothing but sugar, artificial sweeteners, and syrups.

All of these artificial drinks are just weighing us down and pushing us to **lethargy**. This category of drinks is one thing I would eliminate completely.

I tried, I really tried not to be restrictive, but with these particular items I just can't not be. With any liquid you're drinking recognize if there are artificial ingredients in that drink. If there are, you're better off with an alternative. Let's move on to more pleasant conversation.

The motion in the ocean.

The hydration your body craves.

The only reason you're alive right now.

We're talking about **water**.

There are really only three things you truly need to live: a temperate climate, food, and water. Food, you can last quite a while without. Many sources will give you about 30 to 40 days the human body can live without any food. This ***drastically decreases*** without water. You can only survive about 3 to 4 days without water based on the situation.

Water is important for every function in your body. The majority of your body is composed of water. It is the majority component of everything from cells to muscles. With that said, <u>we need lots of it</u>.

Most Americans do not drink enough. A good estimate is to drink about 80 ounces of water daily, a little more if you're very active. This is equivalent to about seven, 12-ounce glasses, or five, 16-ounce water bottles. With water it is extremely hard to become over-hydrated. You would have to drink about 32 ounces of water or more every hour for several hours to accomplish this.

Since it is quite easy to become dehydrated, so we will steer on the side of drinking a little more water and peeing a couple more times per day than drinking too little and having decreased performance and head-aches.

You will have to find the balance of how much water you need daily, but I would stick to about 80 ounces as this is what I have found to be the average amount necessary for most people.

Try infusing your water with fruits, vegetables, and herbs to make it a tasty experience. Putting in a couple mint leaves, a slice or two of cucumber, and a strawberry cut in half can completely change your hydration experience.

Mineral or sparkling waters are fun to throw in the mix as well. Squeeze a slice of lemon or lime in these to up the ante! Always keep water with you and sip it constantly throughout the day. Drinking enough water will help you keep your focus and function at the highest level possible. This is another one of those things that can affect everything from *your work life to your love life*.

Tying in your water consumption with your goals is very realistic, because it really can help you work smarter or keep your love life as passionate and active as possible. If water affects everything in your body, then it affects everything in your life. Don't take it for granted and know it is an *essential part* to creating the life you so long for.

To wrap up the drinks portion of this section: when in doubt, try to drink water constantly throughout the day, as it is the most important thing we need to live, everything else drink in moderation, and eliminate soda or treat it like a delicacy, with rare use.

Key Takeaways:

- **Adequately hydrate yourself throughout the day to maximize your performance in every aspect of life.**

- **Eliminate sodas and artificial drinks.**

- **Everything else drink in moderation.**

- Infuse your water with herbs, fruits, and vegetables to create a delicious hydration experience.

4.14: Developing Your Palate

This is one of the most exciting parts of cooking and exploring nutrition. Unfortunately, in America almost everything we eat is either overly salty or intensely too sweet.

We miss out on many of the subtler flavors ranging from earthy to bitter and everything in-between. There are so many different spices, herbs, and flavors out there, why not explore them all? You might surprise yourself with a new favorite go-to dish.

Pair different oils with different meals.

Mix and match your spices.

The possibilities are endless!

This ties in with treating your cooking and food as a journey. *This is something new and exciting*. Live it to the fullest. Get excited about developing new habits and tastes. Look forward to your meals, explore your tastes, and I promise you this will be a riveting adventure!

Key Takeaways: Read the 135 words above damnit!

4.15: Wrapping it Up

Remember how we were talking about cooking in the psychology section; it can be fun or it can be miserable, it is up to you. Make cooking and your nutrition fun and a priority, and all of your excuses will melt away.

Get excited about your grocery shopping trips with all of the new information you have learned, be an intelligent consumer!

Look at your nutritional habits as helping you accomplish any goal in your life since they directly relate.

Invest in yourself and get a cook book, read some recipes online for a few minutes before you start preparing your meal, and let your imagination run *wild*.

The nutrition section isn't meant to create some harsh guidelines and tell you only to eat these things. With many of the quality suggestions they are just that, <u>suggestions</u>. Eating **whole foods and balancing your nutrition** are always the **first** priority.

I listed out just about all of your basic examples of whole foods above. You can now pick any or all of them that you like. I encourage you to try as many as possible. An easy way to get started on this adventure is to make a grocery list with three categories:

Whole foods you already know you like, that you will buy this week (60-70% of the list):

_____

_____

_____

_____

_____

_____

_____

_____

_____

Whole foods that you're interested in trying (10-20% of the list):

_____

_____

_____

_____

The "bad foods" or "shitty foods" that will fill out the other 20% of

the 80/20 rule:

_____

_____

_____

_____

While doing this try to continue to **balance** your list with

healthy proteins, produce carbohydrates, non-produce

carbohydrates, and good fats. Don't be afraid of new foods or

recipes.

You might not even know if you like something until you use it in a delicious recipe or cook it a certain way. Think of some meals you would like to cook that week before heading to the grocery store or look up recipes online beforehand.

It can't be stressed enough that every single person on this planet is different when it comes to food. The only person who can find out what you like, **is you**. Take control of your food destiny and watch that unicorn you're on giddy up.

Key Takeaways:

- **Find YOUR perfect diet through this journey with exploration!**

- **Eating whole foods and balancing your nutrition are always the first priority with food.**

- **Stick to healthy eating habits and nutrition will soon become intuitive and thought-less.**

Chapter 5: More Than Just an Hour in the Gym

While this is last on the list, physical health is still very important. You can find numerous studies that show a simple common denominator; the larger the circumference of one's waist, the more likely they are to have various diseases and complications.

Not to mention that physical exercise has been shown to improve memory, thinking skills, increase the size of the brain, and even help thwart off terminal illness' like Alzheimer's disease.[47,48] I will finally add that exercise has been shown to help ward off depression and anxiety.[49]

A little activity truly goes a long way in impacting your wealth, health, happiness, and love. Without it, you are certain to come up short in every one of those aspects of your life.

Besides the actual health aspects, we should also talk about the biology and kinesiology of the human body.

Bear with me.

I know we've hit this a couple times, but your kinesiology and biology are so important and really can change the way you view your modern life. With all species, there are normal mechanisms that they should be able to do, ones they have done for a really long time.

If you saw a lion that was so fat, that it could not run the length of a football field, let alone do it quickly, would you think this is normal? Then why do we think this is normal with humans? The human body is meant to be able to do a vast array of movements:

R U N! P U

S S H!

W

I

R O N

L L! G!

!   P

B   U   S   T!

M   L   Q   A

I   L!   U   !

L   P

C   C   R   A   U

              W   L!   M

                         J

We should be able to do all of these actions in a variety of situations. So just because you saw an obese person hip hop dancing on a Facebook video, that doesn't mean that they can move their body the way they are supposed to.

When talking about physical health our joints are a priority. Being overweight causes immense pressure on your joints overtime and eventually leads to replacement surgeries that could otherwise be avoided. While I don't want to dwell on the physical aspect of health we still have to address it, because despite what some may put on the internet being overweight is not healthy.

This **doesn't** mean you should *obsess* over it, but you should understand that you need to change this. In order to lose weight, the best thing you can do is remain active throughout the day, use good nutritional strategies, and practice healthy lifestyle and psychological habits.

An hour at the gym is not going to make a big impact if the rest of your day is a *hodge-podge of bad habits*. This is why we have to look at your health from a psychological, lifestyle, nutritional, and physical perspective. From a physical perspective focus on your overall habits as well as your activity levels throughout the day, not just one workout.

After reading this section you will have the tools to make exercise fun again!

You will no longer dread it, but actually look forward to throwing in some extra fun throughout your day. You don't have to become a gym bro dedicating your life to the iron. You don't have to become CrossFit addicts who are hell bent on telling every person they know their damn workout of the day. You just need to invest a little extra time of your day into having fun while being active.

Key Takeaways:

- **General activity throughout the day will always be more important than an hour at the gym.**

- **Use the amazing body you have in every way to experience all of your capabilities designed by your natural kinesiology.**

5.1: You are Different, Exercise like It

Our world has changed quite a bit in modern times, but if our hunting and gathering ancestors saw us packed into fluorescently lit rooms, sitting on machines, and running on treadmills like gerbils there is no doubt in my mind they would only say, "**What the fuck.**"

I think most of our modern life they would be able to understand.

Planes and cars: "I get it, they can travel very far distances in a short amount of time now."

Cell phones: "Makes sense, now I can text Fred to see if he is ready for our morning hunt, instead of walking in on him and Wilma during boom boom time."

But gyms: "Gyms! *They are like caged animals!*" There's a whole world out there! Fields, trees, bridges, buildings, and parks.

Now, if you love the gym then that is <u>fantastic</u>! You have found your thing whether it be group Zumba classes or lifting weights and that is amazing. Keep doing your thing!

On the contrary, like the majority of people, you may loathe the gym. You may not be a fan of the environment. The activities are torture for you rather than fun. This makes you dread going to the gym and unsuccessful with many fitness programs.

If you are one of these people, you need a change. I've highlighted this a few times throughout this book, but fitness should be natural. Cavemen did not wake and say, "Today, I go 5 mile run run!" No, they did it because it encompassed their lives and survival. Fitness was something much bigger than themselves.

While our ancient ancestors lived in a world of scarcity, we now live in a world of abundance. In our abundant world you can spend your time doing anything, so if you don't like what you are doing it is way too easy to trade it off for something else i.e.

watching TV. In saying this, the first rule of your fitness journey is to choose something you *like*!

I don't care if it's blasting music in your house and dancing, rock climbing, jiu-jitsu, barre, tricking, climbing trees, playing with your infant child, taking walks, yoga, **anything**! The goal is to perform a fun activity that you enjoy a few times a week, which will also keep your activity levels up. Do you want to hear a secret?

All exercise is relatively the same to the body.

The body recognizes movement, the intensity of said movement, and the endurance of this movement. Your body does not know if you're climbing on the side of a mountain or on a tree. Your body only knows what muscles are engaged and what energy system it has to tap into to sustain that activity. The same goes for resistance.

Resistance is resistance!

This pisses gym bros off the most. Most don't understand that if you contract your bicep and flex as hard as you can, this can create the same stimulus as contracting your bicep while lifting a heavy weight. Now if you had a friend pulling your arm back trying to make it straight again, this would be called **resistance**.

The body does not know if the resistance is coming from a 40-pound kettlebell, a 50-pound dumbbell, a 200-pound barbell, or a partner pulling your arm back. The only thing the body realizes is how strong the resistance is and the intensity it has to react too.

That's it.

All of this, "powerlifting is better, no bodybuilding is better, no bodyweight exercise is better," really isn't relevant. The answer to this argument is pretty simple. If you're trying to become competitive in any of those sports whether it be powerlifting or rock climbing, then practice that sport a lot. If you don't care about being competitive, then that argument is pointless and you should simply do what you enjoy. However, there is no "better" exercise, it is only "better" if your goal is to excel in that sport.

With that said, if you are someone who wants to be competitive in any activity then there is a good chance you enjoy it. So dive in, go find your ideal program or routine, it will make a difference - *for that person*.

For anyone else who is just trying to get their health back and use their health as a tool to accomplish their larger goals, then you shouldn't be worrying about becoming the next Arnold Schwarzenegger or competing.

Now the pressure is off!

You ***do not*** need to worry about doing the "*best*" exercise or the "*best fat burning routine*." You ***do not*** need to worry about what will *get you in shape the fastest*.

The paradox of choice has been largely narrowed down to just choosing <u>what you like</u>. Treating this as a journey, just as you did with nutrition, will make it a much more enjoyable experience. Try out lots of different activities! Find your niche!

Don't be discouraged if you tried something and you did not like it. You're one step closer to finding the thing you will like and you would have never known if you liked Zumba or yoga or whatever activity, if you didn't try it.

For me personally, this has been a long journey. I've tried many different activities, and fell in love with many as well, but my favorite of them all has been *movement training*. This kind of exercise isn't about repetitions and sets, it's not about some perfect form or technique, it boils down to something so simple: **movement**.

Movement can be anything from doing a cartwheel, to swinging on a tree, balancing on a curb, running across a grassy field, anything. It can be as advanced as performing an iron cross on the gymnastic rings or as simple as crawling across the floor. Most fitness programs go wrong the same way that diets go wrong: they're restrictive.

It's against human nature to be restricted. We like to spread out everywhere, see new things, and explore every domain possible. Most programs try to sit you down on a bike for 45 minutes exactly with every move pre-planned. They may put you on five different exercise machines, using exactly this weight, for this many repetitions.

This is inherently restrictive.

You are falsely taught that this is how you get results! This is how you lose weight, by only doing these things, this certain way! This is so false and we need to get past it. If you want to be the best cycler in the world, well then yes, you're going to have to cycle and cycle a lot.

Although, what if you don't want to be that?

Key Takeaways:

- **There is no "best" fitness program, focus on finding the activities you enjoy no matter what they are!**

- **You don't have to go to a gym or subscribe to any one program to be healthy, tailor your fitness to your personal needs!**

5.2: Playing Like a Child

For the majority of us it's time to get back to free form fitness.

Earlier in our human history we used fitness as a way of survival,

now it can be used as a form of play.

So contrary to American beliefs: **play**.

You did this everyday as a child, you weren't methodical about

it counting reps and sets and you didn't program or time it, <u>you</u>

<u>simply had fun</u>! You went out to a playground ran around and

climbed everything in sight, you played tag and other fun games,

and you played sports just to play them. Somewhere along the way

while growing up it became a *stigma* to have fun while exercising.

Now we are even trying to stop children from having fun! I

cannot stand it when I hear this argument, "We give trophies to

every five-year-old in the soccer league, they're never taught

winning is a good thing!"

Are you fucking kidding me? Let me explain something....

They.

Are.

Five-year-olds.

They should just be having fun!

There are times to have winners and losers, and there are times to have fun. As children get older and more competitive leagues are available to them, then there's a time for winning and losing. Naturally, more athletic children gravitate towards these competitive leagues and there are try-outs for them.

Until that point arrives it is important to teach children the importance of activity. In a country where our health is a shit-storm epidemic and 70% of the population is obese or overweight, it's <u>pretty damn important</u> we teach kids being active and playing sports is <u>fun</u> and <u>healthy</u>, not just competition.

It has recently been shown through research children who are more physically fit actually *have larger brains and better memories.*[43] With studies like this, we are once again reminded that exercise goes much **deeper** than appearances.

Just as exercise can be used to help children improve in the classroom, exercise can help adults improve in the workforce. Stalled on a report or project? Go run around for a minute, jump towards the sky, crawl on your hands and feet under a tree or do a few good feeling stretches. This will help your productivity much more then looking at an internet site or watching TV. Enough about you, back to the kiddos.

Not only do we try to sway children from having fun, but we lead with a piss poor example. No wonder kids are becoming more and more unhealthy and fat. What do you do after work? Come home, sit on the couch, and watch TV. So what do your children want to do? Get home from school, sit on the couch, and watch TV also.

Do as I say, not as I do, is not a very good way to lead.

What if instead you went outside and played catch with your child. What if you lead by an even better example and played tag with your husband or wife? This would be showing your child that you don't just play because of them, you play because it's enjoyable!

Fun does not have to be a byproduct of a workout.

*Fun can be the **entire mission** of fitness and health.*

Change your mindset to that of a child who can't stand sitting at their desk at the end of a school day, because all they want to do is go outside and play games with their friends. Play games, play on a jungle gym, play with friends, family, and significant others and play sports just to play them. What's the common denominator in all of this? ***Moving***.

That's right, just move. Nothing complicated, no programs, no tracking your every repetition. You can do whatever it is that you want to do as long as you are moving!

Again, if you want 20 inch biceps you'll have to do hypertrophy curls every 2 days. If a 5:00 mile is your goal, you have to run mile repeats and sprints.

There is no doubt about that.

If your goals are getting a smaller midsection, losing weight, and becoming leaner then these smaller changes will come naturally through healthy psychological, lifestyle, and nutritional habits with some small amounts of exercise.

If your goal is not a physical extreme, then it will be accomplished naturally by following the strategies in this book and exercising moderately. Focus on your movement. It does not matter how you move as long as you are moving!

Bodyweight exercise, lifting weights, yoga, walking, doing fun activities like kayaking, as long as you're always doing something active, this is the only thing that matters. If your goal is being mentally, physically, and emotionally healthy while working toward the life you want, *then all you have to do is go get moving*!

Get your family and friends involved to play games. Play all of the fun games you used to when you were growing up like kick the can, hide and seek, or capture the flag. You can even have neighborhood gatherings and the adults can sip alcoholic beverages while playing these games.

Of course if you're drunk, don't blame me if you trip while running toward home-base and face-plant. Although, drinking in moderation and playing these games can be a fun changeup from the usual night out. As my Dad always says, you may even end up beer neutral: (Beers in = Beers Burned) = Beer Neutral.

With the wondrous world of the internet you can always find new and exciting games to play with any number of people. There are how-to videos on YouTube for just about any activity. No matter if your passion is tricking, yoga, or you want to learn easy progressions to a pull-up, it can all be found online.

Focusing on movement will make exercising convenient, as you can literally move anywhere and everywhere. Most of the time people won't work out because they have to go somewhere to do it. Take away that excuse, because with movement you have the entire world from your bedroom to China.

Key Takeaways:

- **Move. That is all you need to do for a physically healthy lifestyle, move in any way you want and focus on having fun while you move!**

- **Make fun the priority and goal of your activity.**

5.3: The Endurance Species

Moving throughout the entire day is *much more important* than an hour of intense exercise. We were created to be endurance animals.

We can't run very fast compared to most animals.

We aren't very strong compared to other species.

We aren't exceptionally tough, either.

We were meant for constant, low impact, low intensity movement: **endurance**. This does not mean that we can't sprint or lift heavy objects when needed, but our bodies were not built for doing *those activities constantly or too often*. Our energy systems prove this. The structure of our musculoskeletal system proves this.

When it comes to fitness, if all you want is to look better and be healthy, then don't be consumed by strict workout programs and exercises you don't enjoy. Do things you enjoy and have the only objective be activity and fun.

Activity doesn't have to be tracked.

It doesn't have to be written down.

It doesn't have to have a time frame.

It just needs to happen in some form or another.

With this freeform way of exercising, there is no pressure. No stress. No torture or forcing yourself to do things you don't enjoy.

Now that you know some ways to make exercising fun again, let's think of a 30-minute-ish time slot you currently fill with mindless activities that can be swapped for some time having fun and being physically active.

Could you swap out 30-minutes of television for playing outside with your children? What about 30-minutes of Xbox for playing sports outside with some friends?

Could you bring an extra pair of clothes to work so you could play at a park nearby for a little while afterwards and avoid the 5:00 traffic jam you'd otherwise be sitting through doing nothing anyway?

List at *least one time* slot of mindless activity you currently

partake in that could be swapped for some fun physical activity.

Activity I Will Swap: Fun Exercise I Will Do Instead:

_____   _____

_____   _____

_____   _____

Stop looking at fitness as a stand-alone product. Make overall

movement be a portion of your lifestyle you work to improve. It is

a piece of your health puzzle for a better life and accomplishing

your goals. This creates more importance and a better

understanding of how exercise really affects your life.

Get your blood pumping, the endorphins flowing, and have

fun! By focusing on fun and activity levels you can truly make

fitness an enjoyable habit, not something you dread. Take control of your fitness and <u>find what is best for you</u>, don't let anyone else tell you what this is.

Key Takeaways:

- **Swap out more periods of your day for small amounts of movement.**

- **Find out what activities you enjoy and stay active, this is the only thing you need to live a physically healthy lifestyle.**

Chapter 6: You're Almost There

If you got to the end of this book and said, "But you didn't tell me how to get rich or give me a step by step guide to getting the girl of my dreams," then you missed the larger lessons and should probably re-read the book.

As with anything in life, there is never any step-by-step guide that is going to get you exactly where you need to go, and if you're expecting one from this then you have much to learn.

If you got to the end and you're saying, "Well that's all pretty much common sense," this may be true. A lot of this book is simple knowledge backed by research, but are you actually performing these actions? Do you react calmly when something bad happens? Have you stepped away from the negativity in your life? Do you regularly destress through breathing exercises? Do you track your lifestyle habits and seek improvement where you're lacking? Do you eat perfectly clean and are you active throughout the entire day? **Most likely no**. Everyone, including myself, has to continually work at these things constantly throughout their life. <u>There is a big difference between knowing something is common sense and performing the actions necessary to change.</u> This is where the strategies, interactions, and implementations of this book come in. It may be common sense, but you needed ways to make these actions habits and to engrain them, so they are no longer common sense, but common actions.

I do hope that as you read through this book you gained practical knowledge. That you're starting to see your health, your mentality, and your habits much differently. You're starting to realize the traps you were caught in before and that the way you were thinking was impeding your life. Health isn't a small goal, but rather something that directly affects every aspect of your life.

None of my rules or principles are quick fixes. You aren't going to read the section on the 80/20 rule or investing in yourself and wake up tomorrow to be a fit millionaire. My desire, is for this book to completely change your actions and thoughts, so as time progresses you're moving your life towards your goals whether knowingly or subconsciously.

If you start thinking about your health differently it will change how you start thinking about the rest of your life. If you start taking actions that will positively affect your health, you will also begin taking actions that positively affect your goals.

When first reading this book it may seem overwhelming.

There are so many suggestions that you don't know where to start. Start by brainstorming and realizing which parts of your health need the most work. Slowly add better psychological, lifestyle, nutritional, and physical principles to your life little by little.

Look back at the interactive sections and see where you need to make changes. Relate everything back to your goals and outline how each change you make, will get you closer to the life you want. Make it fun and get excited about your journey.

I'm going to end this with my favorite quote of all time, by a man who lived a beautiful life. Mahatma Gandhi once said, "Be the change that you wish to see in the world."

I did not write this book to make an exorbitant amount of money, nor did I write this for notoriety. I saw many problems: unhappiness, regret, pain, insecurity, low self-esteem, poor decision making, and I correlated all of these back to health. With my expertise I sought out only one objective: giving back as much value as I possibly could to the largest amount of people across this country.

Your struggle is not unique. I have seen it affect so many people I know personally, from clients to friends and family. It is so wide spread that it truly has become an epidemic and anything I do to help reverse this epidemic *gives me joy and purpose*.

I tried to keep this as short and sweet as possible. I meticulously looked at every sentence and if I thought it wouldn't add value to you as a reader, I cut it. I wanted this to be thought-provoking and demand action.

I truly believe as a society and even as a species, we are only as strong as our weakest links. If we can create a healthy society together, we will enhance our progression as a population. We will become more innovative, advanced, and most importantly, find true happiness in every corner of life.

Diets haven't worked for a majority of the population, nor have workout routines, or other books that lay out the same traditional plans. With my strategies and techniques, I have created an all-encompassing environment that will not only encourage change, but force it.

Decide today that you're going to take control of your health to improve your wealth, happiness, love, and success. Look back at everything you have written down throughout this book and stick to it.

You wrote down those goals for a reason!

You wrote down those changes to implement because you know they are your weak links.

You now have all the tools to maximize your health and make all of your goals come true. With this change in health will come a change in everything else in your life. If you truly create habits with the techniques I have laid out in this book, then anything is possible. Have fun on your journey and always strive for better.

Sincerely,

Garrett Busch

Sources

1.   Yang, Lin and Graham A. Colditz. "Prevalence Of Overweight And Obesity In The United States, 2007-2012". *JAMA Internal Medicine* 175.8 (2015): 1412. Web. 13 Oct. 2016. <http://archinte.jamanetwork.com/article.aspx?articleid=2323411>.

2.   Adkins, Amy. "Majority of U.S. Employees Not Engaged Despite Gains in 2014." *Gallup.com*. Gallup, 28 Jan. 2015. Web. 07 Sept. 2016. <http://www.gallup.com/poll/181289/majority-employees-not-engaged-despite-gains-2014.aspx?utm_source=alert&utm_medium=email&utm_content=heading&utm_campaign=syndication>.

3.   Pratt, Laura A., Ph.D, Debra J. Brody, M.P.H., and Qiuping Gu, M.D. "Antidepressant Use in Persons Aged 12 and Over: United States, 2005–2008." *Centers for Disease Control and Prevention*. Cdc.gov, 19 Oct. 2011. Web. 07 Sept. 2016. <http://www.cdc.gov/nchs/data/databriefs/db76.htm>.

4.   Mayonewsreleases. "Nearly 7 in 10 Americans Take Prescription Drugs, Mayo Clinic, Olmsted Medical Center Find." *Http://newsnetwork.mayoclinic.org*. Mayo Clinic, 19 June 2013. Web. 07 Sept. 2016. <http://newsnetwork.mayoclinic.org/discussion/nearly-7-in-10-americans-take-prescription-drugs-mayo-clinic-olmsted-medical-center-find/>.

5.   Hurley, Dan. "Divorce Rate: It's Not as High as You Think." *The New York Times*. Nytimes.com, 19 Apr. 2005. Web. 07 Sept. 2016. <http://www.nytimes.com/2005/04/19/health/divorce-rate-its-not-as-high-as-you-think.html>.

6.   Ergotron. "New Survey: To Sit or Stand? Almost 70% of Full Time American Workers Hate Sitting, but They Do It All Day Every Day." *New Survey: To Sit or Stand? Almost 70% of Full Time American Workers Hate Sitting, but They Do It*. Ergotron, 17 July 2013. Web. 07 Sept. 2016. <http://www.prnewswire.com/news-releases/new-survey-to-sit-or-stand-almost-70-of-full-time-american-workers-hate-sitting-but-they-do-it-all-day-every-day-215804771.html>.

7.   "Chronic Low Back Pain on the Rise: UNC Study Finds 'alarming Increase' in Prevalence." *UNC School of Medicine*. Med.unc.edu. N.p., 9 Feb. 2009. Web. 07 Sept. 2016. <http://www.med.unc.edu/www/newsarchive/2009/february/chronic-low-back-pain-on-the-rise-unc-study-finds-alarming-increase-in-prevalence>.

8.   "Facts on Chronic Pain." (n.d.): N.p., Middle Tennessee State University. *MTSU.Edu*. Web. 07 Sept. 2016. <http://www.mtsu.edu/healthpro/documents/chronic_pain.pdf>.

9.   "About Chronic Diseases." (n.d.): N.p. National Health Council. *National Health Council.Org.*, 29 July 2014. Web. 07 Sept. 2016. <http://www.nationalhealthcouncil.org/sites/default/files/NHC_Files/Pdf_Files/AboutChronicDisease.pdf>.

10.   Jones, Jeffery M. "In U.S., 40% Get Less Than Recommended Amount of Sleep." *Gallup.com*. Gallup, N.p., 19 Dec. 2013. Web. 07 Sept. 2016. <http://www.gallup.com/poll/166553/less-recommended-amount-sleep.aspx>.

11.   Happify. "90 Percent Of People Say They Have A Major Regret. Here's How To Move Past It." *The Huffington Post*. Happify.com, 26 June 2014. Web. 07 Sept. 2016.

<http://www.huffingtonpost.com/2014/06/26/regret-infographic_n_5529641.html>.

12. Stillman, Jessica. "Complaining Is Terrible for You, According to Science." *Inc.com*. N.p., 29 Feb. 2016. Web. 07 Sept. 2016. <http://www.inc.com/jessica-stillman/complaining-rewires-your-brain-for-negativity-science-says.html>.

13. Bates, Claire. "Is This the World's Happiest Man? Brain Scans Reveal French Monk Has 'abnormally Large Capacity' for Joy - Thanks to Meditation." *Mail Online*. Associated Newspapers, N.p., 31 Oct. 2012. Web. 07 Sept. 2016. <http://www.dailymail.co.uk/health/article-2225634/Is-worlds-happiest-man-Brain-scans-reveal-French-monk-abnormally-large-capacity-joy-meditation.html>.

14. Zmuda., Natalie. "Bottom's Up! A Look at America's Drinking Habits." *Advertising Age News RSS*. AdAge.com, N.p., 27 June 2011. Web. 07 Sept. 2016. <http://adage.com/article/news/consumers-drink-soft-drinks-water-beer/228422/>.

15. "Sleep and Disease Risk." *Division of Sleep Medicine at Harvard Medical School*. WGBH Educational Foundation, N.p., 18 Dec. 2007. Web. 07 Sept. 2016. <http://healthysleep.med.harvard.edu/healthy/matters/consequences/sleep-and-disease-risk>.

16. Tetley, Michael. "Instinctive Sleeping and Resting Postures: An Anthropological and Zoological Approach to Treatment of Low Back and Joint Pain." *BMJ : British Medical Journal* 321.7276 (2000): 1616–1618. Web. 07 Sept. 2016. <http://www.ncbi.nlm.nih.gov/pmc/articles/PMC1119282/>.

17. Doucleff, Michaeleen. "Lost Posture: Why Some Indigenous Cultures May Not Have Back Pain." *NPR.org*. NPR, N.p., 08 June 2015. Web. 07 Sept. 2016. <http://www.npr.org/sections/goatsandsoda/2015/06/08/412314701/lost-posture-why-indigenous-cultures-dont-have-back-pain>.

18. Fahrni, Harry W., and Gordon Trueman. "Comparative Radiological Study of the Spines of a Primitive Population with North Americans and Northern Europeans." *The Journal of Bone and Joint Surgery* 47B.3 (1965): 552-555. *Boneandjoint.org.uk*. Web. 07 Sept. 2016. <http://www.boneandjoint.org.uk/content/jbjsbr/47-B/3/552.full.pdf>.

19. Grabmeier, Jeff. "Study: Body Posture Affects Confidence In Your Own Thoughts." *Resarchnews.osu.edu*. Research Communications The Ohio State University, n.d. Web. 07 Sept. 2016. <http://researchnews.osu.edu/archive/posture.htm>.

20. Link, Erin Lynn. "Is Sitting the New Smoking? - Illinois State University News." *News.illinoisstate,edu*. Illinois State University News, N.p., 24 Nov. 2014. Web. 07 Sept. 2016. <https://news.illinoisstate.edu/2014/11/sitting-new-smoking/>.

21. Owen, N., A. Bauman, and W. Brown. "Too Much Sitting: A Novel and Important Predictor of Chronic Disease Risk?". *British Journal of Sports Medicine* 43.2 (2008): 81-83. Web. 07 Sept. 2016. <http://bjsm.bmj.com/content/43/2/81.full>.

22. Kilbom, A., and T. Brundin. "Circulatory Effects of Isometric Muscle Contractions, Performed Separately and in Combination with Dynamic Exercise." *Eur J Appl Physiol Occup Physiol* 6.36(1) (1976): 7-17. *Pubmed.gov*. Web. 07 Sept. 2016. <http://www.ncbi.nlm.nih.gov/pubmed/1001318>.

23. Hunter, Emily M., and Cindy Wu. "Give Me a Better Break: Choosing Workday Break Activities to Maximize Resource Recovery." *Journal of Applied Psychology* 101(2) (Feb 2016): 302-311. *Psycnet.apa.org*. Web. 07 Sept. 2016. <http://psycnet.apa.org/index.cfm?fa=buy.optionToBuy&id=2015-36861-001>.

24. Seiter, Courtney. "The Science of Breaks at Work: Change Your Thinking About Downtime." *Open.buffer.com*. Buffer, 21 Aug. 2014. Web. 07 Sept. 2016. <https://open.buffer.com/science-taking-breaks-at-work/>.

25. Hölzel, Britta K., James Carmody, Mark Vangel, Christina Congleton, Sita M. Yerramsetti, Tim Gard, and Sara W. Lazar. "Mindfulness Practice Leads to Increases in Regional Brain Gray Matter Density." *Psychiatry research* 191.1 (2011): 36–43. *PMC*. Web. 07 Sept. 2016. <http://www.ncbi.nlm.nih.gov/pmc/articles/PMC3004979/>.

26. Paulus, Martin P., MD. "The Breathing Conundrum – Interoceptive Sensitivity and Anxiety." *Depression and anxiety* 30.4 (2013): 315–320. *PMC*. Web. 07 Sept. 2016. <http://www.ncbi.nlm.nih.gov/pmc/articles/PMC3805119/>.

27. Luders, Eileen, Nicolas Cherbuin, and Florian Kurth. "Forever Young(er): Potential Age-defying Effects of Long-term Meditation on Gray Matter Atrophy." *Front. Psychol.* 5:1551. doi: 10.3389/fpsyg.2014.01551 Web. 07 Sept. 2016. <http://journal.frontiersin.org/article/10.3389/fpsyg.2014.01551/full>.

28. "Practice Makes Perfect, York U Brain Study Confirms." *News.yorku.ca*. York Media Relations, N.p., 29 Jan. 2016. Web. 07

Sept. 2016. <http://news.yorku.ca/2016/01/29/practice-makes-perfect-york-u-brain-study-confirms/>.

29. Miller, Joshua W., Ph.D, Danielle J. Harvey, Ph.D, Laurel A. Beckett, Ph.D, Ralph Green, MD, Sarah Tomaszewski Farias, Ph.D, Bruce R. Reed, Ph.D, John M. Olichney, MD, Dan M. Mungas, Ph.D, and Charles DeCarli, MD. "Vitamin D Status and Rates of Cognitive Decline in a Multiethnic Cohort of Older Adults." *JAMA Neurology* 72.11 (2015): 1295-1303. doi:10.1001/jamaneurol.2015.2115. Web. 07 Sept. 2016. <http://archneur.jamanetwork.com/article.aspx?articleid=2436596>.

30. Kerr, David C.R., David T. Zara, Walter T. Piper, Sarina R. Saturn, Balz Frei, and Adrain F. Gombart. "Associations between Vitamin D Levels and Depressive Symptoms in Healthy Young Adult Women." *Psychiatry Research* 227.1 (30 May 2015): 46-51. http://dx.doi.org/10.1016/j.psychres.2015.02.016. Web. 07 Sept. 2016. <http://www.psy-journal.com/article/S0165-1781(15)00108-0/abstract>.

31. "Olive Oil and Wholegrains 'lower Heart Disease Risk'" *Health News from NHS Choices*. U.S. National Library of Medicine, 29 Sept. 2015. Web. 07 Sept. 2016. <http://www.ncbi.nlm.nih.gov/pubmedhealth/behindtheheadlines/news/2015-09-29-olive-oil-and-wholegrains-lower-heart-disease-risk/>.

32. Simopoulos, AP. "The Importance of the Ratio of Omega-6/omega-3 Essential Fatty Acids." *Biomed Pharmacother*. 56.(8) (Oct 2002): 365-379. Web. 07 Sept. 2016. <http://www.ncbi.nlm.nih.gov/pubmed/12442909>.

33. Caramia, G. "[The Essential Fatty Acids Omega-6 and Omega-3: From Their Discovery to Their Use in Therapy]." *Minerva Pediatr.* 60.(2) (Apr 2008): 219-233. Web. 07 Sept. 2016. <http://www.ncbi.nlm.nih.gov/pubmed/18449139>.

34. Sharper, A. G. "Cardiovascular Studies in the Samburu Tribe of Northern Kenya." *American Heart Journal* 63.(4) (May 1962): 437-442. Web. 07 Sept. 2016. <https://www.researchgate.net/publication/9656375_Cardiovascular_studies_in_the_Samburu_tribe_of_Northern_Kenya>.

35. Gupta, Parul, Bonglee Kim, Sung-Hoon Kim, and Sanjay K. Srivastava. "Molecular Targets of Isothiocyanates in Cancer: Recent Advances." *Molecular nutrition & food research* 58.8 (2014): 1685–1707. *PMC*. Web. 07 Sept. 2016. <http://www.ncbi.nlm.nih.gov/pmc/articles/PMC4122603/>.

36. Wright, Kenneth. "A Week's worth of Camping Synchs Internal Clock to Sunrise and Sunset, CU-Boulder Study Finds." *Colorado.edu*. CU Boulder Today, N.p., 1 Aug. 2013. Web. 07 Sept. 2016. <http://www.colorado.edu/today/2013/08/01/weeks-worth-camping-synchs-internal-clock-sunrise-and-sunset-cu-boulder-study-finds>.

37. Hsu, Christine. "Aging Research: Eat 40 Percent Less, Live 20 Years Longer." *MedicalDaily.com*. Medical Daily, 03 July 2012. Web. 07 Sept. 2016. <http://www.medicaldaily.com/aging-research-eat-40-percent-less-live-20-years-longer-241096>.

38. Sears, AL, M.D. "Eat Less, Live Longer." *Alsearsmd.com*. AL Sears, M.D., N.p., n.d. Web. 07 Sept. 2016. <http://www.alsearsmd.com/2005/10/eat-less-live-longer/>.

39. Wayman, Erin. "Meet the Contenders for Earliest Modern Human." *Smithsonian Magazine*. Smithsonian, N.p., 11 Jan. 2012. Web. 07 Sept. 2016. <http://www.smithsonianmag.com/science-nature/meet-the-contenders-for-earliest-modern-human-17801455/?no-ist>.

40. Omenn, Glbert S., M.D., Gary E. Goodman, M.D., Mark D. Thornquist, Ph.D, John Balmes, Ph.D, Mark R. Cullen, M.D., Andrew Glass, M.D., James P. Keogh, M.D., Frank L. Meyskens, Jr., M.D., Barbara Valanis, Dr.P.H., James H. Williams, Jr., M.D., Scott Barnhart, M.D., and Samuel Hammar, M.D. "Effects of a Combination of Beta Carotene and Vitamin A on Lung Cancer and Cardiovascular Disease — NEJM." *New England Journal of Medicine* 334 (2 May 1996): 1150-1155. DOI: 10.1056/NEJM199605023341802. Web. 07 Sept. 2016. <http://www.nejm.org/doi/full/10.1056/nejm199605023341802#t=article>.

41. Tavani, A., and C. La Vecchia. "Beta-carotene and Risk of Coronary Heart Disease. A Review of Observational and Intervention Studies." *Biomed Pharmacother*. 53.(9) (OCT 1999): 409-416. Web. 07 Sept. 2016. <http://www.ncbi.nlm.nih.gov/pubmed/10554676>.

42. Lindeberg, S., and B. Lundh. "Apparent Absence of Stroke and Ischaemic Heart Disease in a Traditional Melanesian Island: A Clinical Study in Kitava." *J Intern Med*. 233.(3) (Mar 1993): 269-275. Web. 07 Sept. 2016. <http://www.ncbi.nlm.nih.gov/pubmed/8450295>.

43. Trotter, Shane. "It's Time to Reform America's Bad Habit Factories." *BreakingMuscle.com*. Breaking Muscle, N.p., n.d. Web. 07 Sept. 2016. <http://breakingmuscle.com/family-kids/its-time-to-reform-americas-bad-habit-factories>.

44.   Brower, Vicki. "Mind–body Research Moves towards the Mainstream." *EMBO Reports* 7.4 (2006): 358–361. *PMC*. Web. 07 Sept. 2016. <http://www.ncbi.nlm.nih.gov/pmc/articles/PMC1456909/>.

45.   "EWG's Shopper's Guide to Pesticides in Produce." *EWG's 2016 Shopper's Guide to Pesticides in Produce*. EWG, N.p., n.d. Web. 22 Sept. 2016. <https://www.ewg.org/foodnews/>.

46.   Glass, Emily. "The Environmental Impact of GMOs." *One Green Planet*. OneGreenPlanet.org, N.p., 2 Aug. 2013. Web. 22 Sept. 2016. <http://www.onegreenplanet.org/animalsandnature/the-environmental-impact-of-gmos/>.

47.   Godman, Heidi. "Regular Exercise Changes the Brain to Improve Memory, Thinking Skills - Harvard Health Blog." *Harvard Health Blog RSS*. Harvard Health Publications, N.p., 09 Apr. 2014. Web. 22 Sept. 2016. <http://www.health.harvard.edu/blog/regular-exercise-changes-brain-improve-memory-thinking-skills-201404097110>.

48.   ALZinfo.org. "Physical Activity Keeps the Brain Healthy." *ALZinfo.org*. Fischer Center For Alzheimer's Research Foundation, N.p., n.d. Web. 22 Sept. 2016. <https://www.alzinfo.org/articles/physical-activity-brain-healthy/>.

49.   Mayo Clinic Staff. "Depression and Anxiety: Exercise Eases Symptoms." *Mayoclinic.org*. The Mayo Clinic, N.p., 10 Oct. 2014. Web. 22 Sept. 2016. <http://www.mayoclinic.org/diseases-conditions/depression/in-depth/depression-and-exercise/art-20046495>.

50.   Dew, Tom. "Standing Desks Double Productivity (new Study)." *Sit-stand.com*. N.p., 07 July 2016. Web. 22 Sept. 2016. <https://sit-stand.com/blog/20_Standing-Desks-Double-Productivity>.

51.   Murray, Michael, M.D. "7 Little-Known Benefits of Sunlight." *Care2.com*. N.p., 7 July 2013. Web. 22 Sept. 2016. <http://www.care2.com/greenliving/7-little-known-benefits-of-sunlight.html>.

52.   Maffetone, Phil, M.D. "Sunlight: Good For the Eyes as Well as the Brain - Dr. Phil Maffetone." *Philmaffetone.com*. N.p., 29 Apr. 2015. Web. 22 Sept. 2016. <https://philmaffetone.com/sun-and-brain/>.

53.   Beck, Julie. "Less Than 3 Percent of Americans Live a 'Healthy Lifestyle'." *The Atlantic*. Atlantic Media Company, N.p., 23 Mar. 2016. Web. 22 Sept. 2016. <http://www.theatlantic.com/health/archive/2016/03/less-than-3-percent-of-americans-live-a-healthy-lifestyle/475065/>.

54.   Yousef, Rama. "Giving the Mind a Break Increases Knowledge Retention - The Daily Cougar." *The Daily Cougar*. N.p., 21 Aug. 2014. Web. 03 Oct. 2016. <http://thedailycougar.com/2014/08/21/giving-mind-break-increases-knowledge-retention/>.

55.   *Munro, Dan.* "U.S. Healthcare Spending On Track To Hit $10,000 Per Person This Year". *Forbes.com*. N.p., 4 Jan. 2015. Web. 13 Oct. 2016. <http://www.forbes.com/sites/danmunro/2015/01/04/u-s-healthcare-spending-on-track-to-hit-10000-per-person-this-year/#4784b150294c>.